WINTER SOULSTICE

Celebrating the Spirituality
of the Wisdom Years

JOHN KILLINGER

A Crossroad Book
The Crossroad Publishing Company
New York

The Crossroad Publishing Company
16 Penn Plaza – 481 Eighth Avenue, Suite 1550
New York, NY 10001

Printed in the United States of America

The text of this book is set in 11/16 Goudy Old Style.
The display faces are Goudy Handtooled, Serlio, Minion, and Nofret.

Printed in the United States of America

Killinger, John.
    Winter soulstice : celebrating the spirituality of the wisdom years /
John Killinger.
        p.   cm.
    Includes bibliographical references.
    ISBN 0-8245-2316-4 (alk. paper)
    1. Older Christians – Religious life. 2. Aging – Religious aspects –
Christianity.   I. Title.
BV4580.K55 2005
248.8′5 – dc22

                                                              2005019398

1   2   3   4   5   6   7   8   9   10   10   09   08   07   06   05

For
ANNIE
my dear, beautiful wife for more than half a century
and
ERIC and KRISTER
our two wonderful and incredibly gifted sons
and
PIA and ANGELA
their delightful, adoring wives
and
ELLIE AND CHLOE
our very, very special grandchildren

This is the greatest gift God can give you:
to understand what happened in your life.
To have it explained.
It is the peace you have been searching for.

—Mitch Albom, from
The Five People You Meet in Heaven

Contents

Introduction

I did not intend, when I began writing this book, to make it as autobiographical as it is. I had in mind instead to fashion it around the idea of the title, which is that we can understand the notion of the soul more easily in our elder years than we did when we were young. I wanted to illustrate the way the different aspects of our lives — our memories, ambitions, work, conflicts, even our sexuality — converge in our latter years to produce a unified being and reveal to us what it means to be truly spiritual.

But as I wrote I found myself inevitably turning to my own experience for illustrations. That, I suppose, was natural. After all, who did I know better than myself? In a way it was funny, because most of my life as a teacher and a minister I attempted to keep personal illustrations to a minimum, not wishing my lectures or sermons to be about me. Even then I didn't always succeed. But neither did I fail as egregiously as I have in this book.

After a chapter and a half of writing I looked over the material and said, "This will never do. I must go back, tear it up, and begin again." But as I thought about how I would do that, I realized how important it was that I let the material stand as it was and write the remainder of the book from the same autobiographical point of view.

It was essential, I felt, to keep my thoughts and the elements of my biography together, for in reality each helped to produce the other. If I had not thought as I did, I would not have lived as I did; and if I had not lived as I did, my thoughts would have been very different. The two have always been naturally intertwined.

I apologize to the reader, therefore, if this book appears to be too much about the writer. The truth is that it is not really about me at all. It is actually about the idea it advances — that in our elder years everything about us, our stored memories and experiences, our choices and failures to choose, our friendships and associations, all come together like the tributaries of a river to form the spiritual beings into which we have evolved.

I invite the reader to replace my experiences with his or her own — to say, "Ah, this helps me to understand why I feel this way about such and such. If I only substitute what happened to me on this or that occasion, I find that I come to similar conclusions. And they are conclusions that truly encourage me to feel good about my life and, in turn, to feel good about God, who has been bound up, more fully than I ever realized, with the way I have lived my life."

If this happens, dear reader, it is what I intended.

One

Remembrance of Things Present

Old age is haunted territory. The ghosts of all our experiences converge upon us, drifting in and out like merry wraiths at a convention of specters. The older we become, the more of these ghosts there are and the more easily they appear to come and go. Some days we can't get anything done for watching and listening to them.

I once heard William Maxwell, the writer, say that becoming an old man was the most interesting thing that ever happened to him. I understand that. It *is* interesting, and on my best days I can celebrate it. Then, I can say I wouldn't want to be young again, facing all that unbridled passion and all the bad decisions I had yet to make along my way.

But there are other days when I tend to agree with the figures in Homer's *Iliad* — I know Homer may not have written the *Iliad,* but if he didn't write it, somebody using his name must have done it — that dying is to become a mere shadow of your former self, a little like the fifth or sixth carbon copy in the days when that was the only way to replicate writing on the typewriter (my simile, not Homer's). Heavens, you don't have to wait until you die for that to happen. It starts occurring while you're still alive. I'm already feeling shadowy, a mere wisp of who I was when I was young and ignorant and full of confidence.

It's a funny thing, but the older I get, the more ghosts there are from my earliest life. One night recently I revisited the room where I slept as an infant. I could see every detail of that white wrought-iron crib I was put in every afternoon and night until I was three or four years old. I hadn't thought about it for ages — not in all my life, I believe — and yet here I was, observing its every detail, from the curlicues on certain bars to the way the disappearing side was fastened to the ends when it was raised. I remembered how imprisoned I always felt when I awoke and there was no one in the room to help me out of it.

And then I saw my mother's bed a few steps away, a huge old brass blunderbuss painted the color of red wine, and felt what it was like, when I became old enough, to pry the great hollow caps off the tops of the posts, speak down into the tubes, and hear my voice echo as if I were hallo-ing into a cave. I hadn't revisited that either. Not once since I was a child.

This sent me off on a train of thoughts. My mother and father slept in separate bedrooms — by my father's choice, I am certain. Even as a child, I felt vaguely disturbed by this, for it confirmed my sense that my parents didn't get along. My father, an agricultural agent, was very lean and handsome then, and dressed impeccably in well-cut suits and neatly tailored ties. He looked like a dandy out of a fashionable men's magazine. Women were always turning to look at him. Mother was quite attractive too, with a pretty face and curly brown hair, but her clothes were older and less glamorous, as my father seldom gave her money to buy anything.

Sometimes she would bundle us children up — I had a baby sister two years younger than I — and take us down to father's office to ask for a quarter so she could buy us all a treat at the drugstore. The office was always bustling with farmers, junior ag workers, and smart young secretaries clacking around in high-heel shoes. Almost invariably, we had to wait before seeing my father, who was of course the most important person in the domain. I think he liked the picture it created to have his pretty wife and dressed-up little children coming in to ask for money. Sometimes he behaved teasingly, as if he didn't know whether he had a quarter in his pocket. The secretaries would titter at this, and I was embarrassed for my mother. Even then I wondered why she had no money of her own, but had to come to my father in supplication.

I recalled the cool marble counter of the soda fountain at Coleman's Drug Store, the leather-bottomed stools that stood proudly in front of it, the little collection of tea tables with spring-backed chairs around them, and the pungent odor of medicines and chemicals mixing with the smell of pine cleaner from the old wooden floor. Mother usually got a soda, one of the old-fashioned kind made by putting two scoops of vanilla ice cream and a few squirts of chocolate syrup in the bottom of a tall glass, then spewing carbonated water on it until the glass was brimming with frothy tan liquid. Mr. Coleman himself usually made it, as he seldom had any help in the store. We would sit at one of the small tables, in the old-fashioned chairs, and he would take our order and bring us what we asked for. We children were free to choose between a Coke and a candy bar, each of which cost five cents. I always chose the candy — one of the big Hershey bars whose little squares I broke apart and stacked before eating them — because Cokes tasted too strong and tickled my nose. My sister, Jo, usually wanted a Coke.

Another time, I remembered the time our family went on a picnic outing with father's secretaries and their families to Hall's Gap, a prominent geological feature six or seven miles from Stanford, Kentucky, the small town where we lived. The land approaching Hall's Gap seemed relatively flat and uninteresting, and then suddenly began to rise precipitously, cresting several hundred feet higher in another plateau. The summit of Hall's Gap was attained via a narrow winding road that snaked tortuously back and forth up the side of the mountain. The old farm vehicles, automobiles, and heavily loaded trucks had to labor mightily in the ascent, and people considered the drive both thrilling and scary, especially when they were coming down and their tires squealed on the hairpin curves. The occasional Greyhound buses that made the trip seemed to wheeze and cough on the way up, and sometimes overheated and had to be rested in a pull-off before renewing their attack.

Somewhere on the summit of Hall's Gap, which I'm sure was named by pioneer settlers first making their way into the Kentucky Territory, there stood a fire tower where visitors were permitted to climb several flights of stairs to an even more commanding view, for then they could see well over the tops of the trees that covered the hill. I was not allowed to go up the stairs, as I was only three or four, so my parents left me in the care of a lovely redheaded secretary named Joyce Sandidge. I cannot believe I remember her name after all those years, but that is what it was. Joyce had been up on the tower before and volunteered to keep my sister and me at the bottom while the others went up. She was a sweet woman, but I recall my boyish resentment that I couldn't go up and see the view everyone else was entitled to see.

I recalled two other memories from those years. One was of the day my mother was crossing our street, Danville Avenue, to return a bowl to our neighbor, Mrs. Cullip, a heavy woman with a pleasant, well-modulated voice who always smelled of perfumed soap and dressed in freshly laundered frocks with a lot of flowers on them. Something happened as mother was stepping up onto the high curb in front of Mrs. Cullip's house and she fell, splitting her shin open to the bone. Blood spattered everywhere, even onto the white bowl she managed to save from destruction before handing it to me. She turned and hobbled back to our house in enormous pain. Mrs. Cullip, who had seen everything from her porch, immediately called the town physician, old Dr. Southard. He was at our house in minutes, recleansing the wound (my mother had already washed it), sprinkling it with some kind of powder, and then binding it with gauze. I knew it was a serious wound if my mother, who always cared for my cuts and scratches, could not attend to it herself.

The other memory was of the day when my mother and father had an awful row because she had given him a ring for his birthday and he didn't like it. It was a beautiful gold ring, with what I thought was an absolutely huge ruby in its crown. I knew my mother had saved bits of money for years to get it — money her own father had given her, to which she had added a nickel or dime here and there from the small allowances my father had given us for the drugstore. But my father's remark when my mother gave it to him was cutting: "Why did you do that? The girls at the office were going to buy me a ring." His face betrayed his disappointment. It was a supreme insult to Mother's love, especially as she knew by this time that my father was sweet on one of the girls, a dark-headed woman named Vera. She wept long and bitterly, and I tried to lessen her pain by fetching my old metal bank with a clock face that was supposed to tell how much money was in it, though it didn't work, and offering her my own pennies and nickels as repayment for the unwanted ring. This must have impressed her mightily, for although she didn't cease crying she mentioned it years later and said what a good son I had been.

Seeing the ghost of Vera led me to another time in my youth. We were living in Somerset, Kentucky, then, thirty-six miles from Stanford. It was during World War II, and my father had been appointed manager of the federal employment agency in that prosperous county-seat town. After a year in a large old rental house, he had discovered a small farm for sale a mile or two out of town, with a little brick house on it. He borrowed the money to buy it, the first property he and mother ever owned. The highway that ran in front of our home made a sharp turn at the bottom of a rather long hill, where the road crossed a bridge over a small creek. Motorists enjoying coasting down the hill often panicked when they realized that they might lose control of their vehicles and strike the bridge. There had been a rain in the night and an eighteen-wheeler filled with soda crackers had run into the bridge, scattering boxes of crackers everywhere.

By this time my mother had begun working to supplement the family income, first as a tax accountant during income-tax season and then as the first female agent for the State Farm Mutual Automobile Insurance Company in Kentucky. After school each day, my sister and I sat in her office until she closed and went home to prepare dinner. But it was now summer, and Jo and I were both left at home to look after ourselves. As I was almost twelve and my sister not quite ten, I was nominally in charge.

The morning the cracker truck crashed below our house, our hill, normally quiet except for occasional cars going by, was humming with activity — sheriff's vehicles, wreckers, authorities from the trucking line, and sightseers. Deciding to investigate, Jo and I walked down the road, careful to keep to the side, behind the guardrail. We found large cartons of crackers scattered everywhere, some on the edge of our property. Regarding it as booty, we rescued three or four boxes and stacked them behind the rail.

One of the men from the trucking company, guessing that we were from the nearby house, asked if we had a phone. I said yes and he wanted to know if he might use it. I had locked the house when we left, so would have to return with him. I told Jo to remain exactly where she was, and not to move on any account. Then I walked up the road with the man.

He was a small, slightly built man, wore a tie, a felt hat, and a trench coat, and was very kind and respectful. He was coughing and wheezing and blowing his nose, and it was obvious that he was suffering from a cold, a condition not helped by the drizzling rain. He made his call to headquarters, and I prepared him a drink that my father often made when he had a cold, consisting of lemon juice, water, and an Alka-Seltzer tablet.

When we went back down the hill Jo was not at her post. I realized almost instantly that she had ventured across the road, and guessed that she was somewhere behind the vast pile of cracker boxes on the other side. An air about the men around the wreck, however, conveyed the unmistakable impression that something terrible had happened. No one said anything or moved to stop me as I went over to the boxes and walked behind them. I don't think I had noticed that there was now another vehicle present, a battered old truck with its nose edged into the disheveled cartons. The driver of the truck had been coming down the hill from the opposite direction, applied his brakes, which didn't hold, and plowed into the mountain of boxes. Jo had been standing behind them and the edge of the truck bed caught her in the temple, instantly killing her. I found her lying lifeless among the boxes, her pale face and short blond hair aureoled in blood.

Even now, as I write this, I see her as clearly as I did that day under the misting rain. I had only one impulse: to get back to the telephone and call my parents. Blindly I mounted the hill and let myself into the strangely hollow house. I fumbled with the old rotary phone, dialing my father's office. "Dad," I said, "you'd better get mother and come home. Jo's been hurt. She was hit by a truck." I don't remember that he offered a reply, but I knew he would be there quickly. Instinctively, I returned to the scene of her death for one more look. Then I came back partway up the hill to our garage, a little white building near the road that had once been a small country store, and waited for my parents.

I wish I could take back the first words I spoke when they rolled into the parking space and leapt out to run down the hill. "You'd better not go down there," I said. "She's already dead." My mother uttered a small, inchoate scream as they hurried down the road, my father's arm around her in a shielding, supportive posture I had never before witnessed. I waited at the garage. It was only moments before they returned, father almost carrying mother along. I followed them into the house, where he laid her on the old-fashioned leather studio couch in our dining room. As he went to get her a glass of water, I sat beside her and tried to offer comfort — something I would continue to do for the next several days.

It wasn't long until our house was teeming with people — the minister from the Methodist church (the Baptist church my mother attended was presently without a pastor), a couple of secretaries and an assistant from Dad's office, neighbors, a close friend of my mother's named Erdean Henson. Soon ladies from my mother's Sunday school class began bustling in, bearing platters of cold cuts, potato salad, bread, and desserts of every description. Everyone spoke in hushed tones and appeared very solicitous. Mother wept through most of the greetings they offered, and the women all hugged her. The men mostly appeared awkward and didn't know what to say. My father behaved with quiet dignity through the whole affair, hovering when he needed to hover and speaking when it was called for.

One of my most redemptive memories of this whole experience occurred the day of my sister's funeral. The house was full of people, and I answered a knock at the front door. It was the man who drove the rattletrap truck that killed my sister. He said he would have come sooner but had just been released from jail. Dark stubble covered his chin. He shifted uneasily from side to side, fondling the worn, sweat-stained, disfigured old felt hat in his hands. He asked to see my father. Visions of an altercation flashed through my head as I told Dad who it was and he left whoever he was talking with to go to the front door. Irresistibly, I followed him onto the porch.

The man, whose tattered overalls marked him for a poor farmer, shifted nervously a couple of times and extended his hand to my father, saying how sorry he was and how hurt he knew my folks must be. I had never seen in my father the quality that came through at this crucial moment. He took the man's hand and replied, "I bear no malice." It was curiously stilted speech for my father, yet classic in its simplicity. I have always admired him for that single moment of generosity. Greatly relieved, the man nodded, put the old hat on his head, and walked away.

The Methodist minister, a lean, bespectacled, ascetic-looking man named Dr. Floyd Rose, conducted Jo's funeral in the Baptist church, which was obviously my mother's preference. I remember how beautiful and serene my sister looked in the open coffin at the front of the sanctuary. I recall two other things about the service. One was the minister's lisping speech and his frequent mention of "Ze-sus" — never "Jesus," always "Ze-sus." The other was my father's weeping. I had never before seen him weep.

Three or four months later, in the early fall, I came home from school one afternoon to find my parents already home, which was extremely unusual. Not only that, they had a guest, which was equally unusual. It was Vera, the secretary from my father's old office. I entered in the middle of a discussion. My father had apparently asked my mother for a divorce, saying he wanted to marry Vera. Vera was silent. I don't know if she had spoken before I arrived. Mother said that she loved my father as much as she ever had and would not consent. Dad called her a "dog in the manger" and berated her for trying to hold him. I knew even then that the only thing constraining him was a lack of finances. He wanted mother to return to her father's house and for me to be sent to military school. He simply didn't earn enough money to pay mother alimony, and probably didn't have enough to hire a lawyer if she contested the divorce. The air of the room was oppressively tense.

Perhaps to relieve the tension, my father ordered my mother to go milk the goats. We had a small herd of Nurenbergs and Toggenburgs, and sold goat's milk to several customers who believed it was therapeutic for ulcers and other stomach disorders. Mother was never strong enough to refuse to do as he demanded, so she put on her jacket and headed for the barn, where the goats were already bleating for their dinners. I said I would help, partly because I wished to support her and partly because I didn't want to remain in the room with my father and "that woman." Mother cried all the way to the barn. I helped by scouring the enameled pans and filling them with feed while she nestled against the comforting warmth of the nannies and tugged at their udders until they were empty.

Mother never agreed to a divorce, and for several years my father quit work at noon every Saturday, dressed up, and drove thirty-six miles to Stanford to see Vera, returning about midnight. Mother was very stoic about it, and I often seethed inside at his infidelity, not only to my mother but to our family as a whole. I don't think adults who are engaged in adulterous relationships really stop to consider the enormity of their offense in the hearts of their children.

❧

You see what I mean about the ghosts. By the time we get older, our memories literally teem with them, and they revisit us in the oddest ways and at the strangest times. Often it is in the night, when we waken and can't get back to sleep. The doors of the ballroom are wide open then, and they waltz in and out with incredible freedom, mocking all efforts to banish them.

A lot of fun is made of older people's failing memories, especially their inability to remember names. I don't think it's failing memory at all. I believe our minds are like computers, the finest that ever existed, and just as computers become slow and cranky when their memories are filled with too much data, our minds, when they become crowded with people and events from our pasts, slow down and sometimes balk at delivering information on demand.

The wonderful thing about all these memories is the way they have enlarged our souls. The word "soul" in Hebrew is *nephesh,* a word rich in meanings and associations. While we tend to think of our souls as discrete entities, with boundaries that stop at the edge of our own consciousness, the ancient Hebrews didn't think that way at all. For them the *nephesh* was more like a magnetic field whose edges are ill defined and whose composition merely fades away with distance from the center. It includes not only our own being but the beings of all those closely related to us, especially our families. It also includes our pets or livestock and our other property. A person's soul, among the Hebrews, was understood to become weak when it was deprived of its ancillary beings, all the people and animals and other chattel, and to be strong when it enjoyed a large family and prosperity in all its household. This is a central aspect of the narrative of Job, the legendary figure who lost everything — flocks, herds, children, even his health — and sank into spiritual despondency before God showed mercy and restored him by giving him a new family and even greater wealth than he had before. The figure of Job on the ash heap, scraping his boils with a potsherd, is one of a man deprived of everything that constituted a strong *nephesh.* His restoration was a gift from God because he was entirely too decimated to recover on his own.

When we begin connecting the dots of all the memories we have — a whole lifetime of them — we begin to have a new feeling for the strength and wholeness of our souls. All of life seems to coalesce in who we are now. And even though our physical powers may be waning, we sense a compensating psychic or spiritual power unlike anything we enjoyed when we were young. I have lain in bed with the flu, reduced to a feverish, quivering mass of flesh and bone with absolutely no will to move or get up, yet felt an exquisite satisfaction in the free flow of memories and thoughts flooding through my being, a tidal wave of mental stimulation and connections that actually made me suspect I was fairly glowing with spiritual health and well-being.

Life is a lot more than mere physical strength and prowess. It is a compounding of all that we are, including our experiences and recollections, familial and friendly associations, knowledge of literature and the arts, and spiritual understanding and connection with the core of all existence, whether we name that core God, Allah, Manitou, the First Cause, or the Supreme Being. Most people don't realize how important this is until they become older and find their own *mana,* or personal power, waning. Then they are more prepared to submit to the general power in the cosmos, the transcendent being that is like the sun in our universe, sharing its life and transformative grace with everything.

I was lucky that I felt a calling to Christian ministry when I was an adolescent and therefore spent more time than most people I knew in various kinds of spiritual training. But I nevertheless feel apologetic that for years I expended too much of my energy fulfilling professional expectations and gratifying personal ambitions, with the result that I did not achieve the rarefied level of insight and gratification I might have known. I understood about these things, but I simply did not pursue the life of the soul with the kind of devotion and vigor it deserves. The beautiful thing about growing older is that now I am automatically discovering the bliss of soulfulness. Retirement, which brings a relief from pressing obligations, whispers to my heart that now it is really time to concentrate on the unification of all my being and enjoy my life's final years to the utmost.

The winter "soulstice," as I call it, is a wonderful time for preparing to die. That may sound morbid, but it isn't, especially if one believes, as I do, that death is merely the moment of our graduation from one level of life to another. Our culture has unfortunately lost its ability to look beyond itself to the wider world of the spirit and to anticipate the unspeakable delight of being freed from the flesh and enabled to be and know and love at a higher plane than we have ever experienced. True seekers realize, of course, that this present life is not the final one. There is implanted in their souls a sense of anticipation that carries them far beyond the evidences of their physical senses in this world. They hear whispers of something beyond, and occasionally yield to little shudders of the heart that convince them of a reality far greater than the one we all know in everyday life.

Most people look forward to their retirement years as a time to do the things they always wanted to do but didn't have time for — taking trips, reading great books, learning to cook gourmet dishes, working on their genealogies, even going scuba diving or white-water rafting. Why shouldn't it also be a time for adventures in the spiritual life, for exploring the edges of mystery that border on our ordinary world? I know people who have spent time in monasteries after retiring, or taken up the study of world religions, or become fascinated with psychic phenomena. They understood what old age is really about.

The human soul, when given any attention at all, continues to deepen and expand throughout our lives, and is more capable of enjoying existence in our latter years than in the former. A society that disregards older citizens merely because they're old is shallow and short-sighted. We are more capable of knowing, loving, teaching, and enjoying in our elder years than we ever were before.

⌒ᴐ

But the soul does require working at. The work isn't hard, but it needs to be seen for what it is, a way of developing the soul into an instrument of finer sensitivity and understanding. The thing that really constitutes it is paying attention. It isn't simply a matter of studying or making a journey or engaging in some special activity. No, the work begins with noticing, with being present to your own life and history and feelings, with really concentrating on who you are and what your soul is about.

The thing is, each of us is an inimitable, unrepeatable concatenation of atoms and experience, and nobody else has ever known things precisely the way we can know them or has been exactly who we can be. The soul has its own print, just the way the fingers do. Our job is to discern that print, to begin to compare notes and records in order to find out who we are and what our souls are really like. We can begin the task early, if we are especially sensitive individuals. But we *must* begin it later, if we haven't done so earlier, for it is the greatest work of our elder years, to learn who we are and how everything that has happened to us fits together to create our uniqueness and unrepeatableness. We do it by noticing, by reviewing the signs by which we have arrived at this point of the journey, by seeing how everything fits together. We do it by paying attention to our dreams, reliving our stories, matching up the disparate parts, celebrating our distinctiveness, loving our selves.

Yes, loving our selves is important. We have always thought of love as something that flows out to others, but the way we think of ourselves is also important. Perhaps this is why Jesus said we should love others as we love ourselves — we can't truly and fully love other people until we accept who we are and celebrate that. The medieval mystic Bernard of Clairvaux, in his famous "Ladder of Love," said we begin by loving self for self's sake. Next, we love self for God's sake. Then we love God for God's sake. And finally, when we reach the apex of our existence, we learn to love ourselves for God's sake. But we can't do this until all our baggage is sorted and we know who it is we are loving. Then the love happens without any prompting; it suddenly manifests itself as the natural response to what we have discovered, that we are the centers of something divine, souls cherished by God the way a child is cherished by the mother who has just borne it. When that happens, we are suddenly at peace with the whole world, with everything that is, and we realize that we are actually part of God.

Two

A Matter of Choice

I normally don't spend much time playing "What if...?" But once in a while, when I'm feeling whimsical, I indulge myself. What if I had become an artist, as I once intended, and not a minister? What if I hadn't married the person I married? What if we'd hit a snag in our relationship, as many married people do, and become divorced? What if I hadn't gone to this school or that? What if I had taken one of the many jobs I didn't take? What if I'd never written a book? What if I hadn't started this one?

I'm usually soaking in the tub when I ponder these questions, my mind drifting in and out of the steam, my mood slightly lazy and unfocused. What if I weren't the person I am? Could I have been different, even if I had wished to? Some psychologists and sociologists think our choices largely determine who we become. Others think there is a kind of inevitability about our destinies and the choices don't always make a difference.

Personally, I'm pretty sure my life is largely bound up with the choices I've made across the years, and that now, in the rosy era of my gathering twilight, I need to own those choices as part of my soul in order to know who I really am and make my final preparations for whatever existence lies beyond this one.

My wife has always said I didn't like to make decisions, and that I could never divorce her because by the time I'd made up my mind to do it she wouldn't be around anyway. She was amazed once when I bought a house, the one we live in now, twenty minutes after we had entered it with the Realtor — so amazed, in fact, that her head began to spin and she sat on the stairs and asked, "Do you really know what you're doing?" She was right to wonder, because she is correct; I don't usually make choices quickly.

Maybe this fact makes the major choices in my life all the more pivotal, so that I must pay attention to them now in order to understand myself and my pilgrimage.

෴

The most pivotal choice I ever made was to become a minister. My whole life would have been vastly different if I had gone to art school and become an illustrator, as I envisioned doing when I was enthralled by the paintings of Norman Rockwell, Ben Stahl, and other great *Saturday Evening Post* artists. Even after I began to suspect that God was messing around with my plans — my friend Ernest Campbell used to say that God is always throwing his hat on our Scrabble boards — I tried to stall him because I really saw myself as an artist. I said, "Why can't I be an artist and teach Sunday school classes on the weekend?"

But God was relentless, and knew better than I did what I ought to do with my life.

In the summer of my sixteenth year, I spent a week at Clearcreek, a church camp in the rough, verdant mountains near Pineville, Kentucky. It was meant to be a kind of spiritual adventure, learning experience, and vacation all rolled into one, although I was too young at that point to deserve a vacation, a luxury I don't think my parents had ever enjoyed.

I had been there once before, as a boy of twelve, with a group of so-called Royal Ambassadors from our church — Boy Scouts without uniforms and knot-tying skills. That was in 1945, when World War II, though just ended, was still an excuse for the refectory to serve powdered eggs, reconstituted potatoes, and other culinary delights of the rations era. I hated it the first time around, and wonder that I agreed to return. But this time I was interested in girls, and I knew lots of them would be there.

This time, I thoroughly enjoyed everything about it. There *were* a lot of girls. I was also old enough to appreciate the icy mountain streams, the cool early morning air, the crowds of happy people, and the daily religious services. And I really liked the preacher of the week, a tautly built, middle-aged man from Little Rock, Arkansas, named W. O. Vaught. Dr. Vaught had a kind of masculinity that extended to his sermons, and I found that very attractive. He even got out on the roughly manicured ball field in the afternoons and played softball with us, displaying a healthy swing and a better-than-average ability to run the bases.

Something about all of it — the setting, the ball games, the girls, the religious services — worked its magic on me. One day when the preacher extended a call during the final hymn for those who would follow Jesus in special vocations to come forward, I knew I was being called into ministry and needed to go forward and say so. I didn't hear a special voice or anything like that. I simply knew and responded.

My whole life changed that day. It was the first really big decision I had ever made, and it was a doozy. It changed everything. But I never considered turning back. My life had taken a new direction. Period. No backtracking, no rethinking, no regrets.

My second big decision was the choice of a school. I had intended, before decision number one, to go to art school in Cincinnati, Ohio. Now I knew I would need to go to college or university, and then possibly on to seminary. W. O. Vaught, the minister at Clearcreek, wore a Baylor University T-shirt when he played softball with us. It looked impressive on his trim, muscular torso. I asked him, when I realized how close I was to changing my career objective, if he had gone to Baylor. He said yes, and added that Baylor was "the biggest Baptist school in the world." So when I decided to go into the ministry I elected at the same time to go to Baylor, assuming as I did that Baptists had a natural franchise on Christianity.

During my senior year of high school, the University of Kentucky summoned me to its campus with fourteen other students and offered me a four-year scholarship that would have paid all my expenses plus spending-money. It wasn't even a temptation. I figured God was big enough to take care of me in Texas, although at that time I had only about seven hundred and fifty dollars in the bank and my father had said, when I announced I was going into the ministry, that I could expect no help from him.

I'll never forget the day I arrived in Waco, Texas, to begin my college adventure. I couldn't afford to stay in a dormitory, so I had written to Dr. John Newport, a Baylor professor whose name W. O. Vaught had given me, and asked help in finding lodging off-campus. He sent me the name of a widowed lady who rented rooms, and I wrote her to request a place. She wrote back to say that the rent would be fifteen dollars a month, and I sent her a money order by return mail.

A lady chiropractor in Lenox, Iowa, Dr. Mable Wintermute, learning from my Aunt Lulu that I was going to become a minister, sent me a check for fifty dollars with instructions that I was to fly to Waco when I went. When I arrived at the widow's house from the airport, long after dark, I was disappointed to see what a shabby, rundown place it was. The widow, a sad-looking, unkempt woman, answered the door in an old chenille housecoat. She was smoking a cigarette and coughing. Conducting me to a dark, depressing room with two bunk beds, one under the only window and the other against a wall, she told me to take whichever I liked, as my roommate wouldn't be there until the following day. Neither bed had been made up, and the mattresses were old, lumpy, and soiled.

Then she led me down an equally dark and dismal hallway to show me the bathroom, a smelly little closet with a small sink, a rusty old tub, and a stained commode with a cracked wooden seat. She said if I would wait a minute she would find me a towel and washcloth. I would have to provide these for myself but she would loan me some until I unpacked and found my own.

I had eaten nothing but a sandwich since early morning, and asked where I might find a restaurant. My new landlady said there was a drug-store across the street that served hamburgers and hot dogs until ten. It was already nine-thirty, so I hurried off. Sitting at the counter and eating an overcooked hamburger and some extremely stale potato chips, I felt as desolate as a child lost at the World's Fair. If I could have gotten on a plane and started home that very night, I'm sure I would have done it.

As it turned out, my first year at Baylor exhausted my bank account. So I returned to Kentucky to take stock of my situation. An old minister I knew, W. W. McAlpin, whom everybody called "Brother Mac," was retiring from his work at the Bronston Baptist Church, a small, rural parish ten miles from my home town. Brother Mac asked if I would be interested in assuming his pastorate. I was only eighteen years old and should have demurred. But the job seemed heaven-sent. I could transfer my credits to Georgetown College, the senior Baptist school in Kentucky, and continue my education while earning a living.

The church agreed, because they loved Brother Mac and he assured them that I was smart and would do a good job. So at eighteen I was ordained and became the minister of my first parish. It was a fateful turn of events, for not only did I do a reasonably good job the first time out of the stall but being the minister of that little church led to my marrying the girl I did.

When I began my ministry at Bronston Baptist Church, the church had no pianist. So I asked Anne Waddle, a talented young musician from my home church, to accompany me each Sunday and play for the services. I had written to Anne a few times while I was at Baylor and had dated her when I was home for Christmas. Now, in this new situation, our relationship deepened considerably, and three months into it, in December, I presented her with an engagement ring. We were driving to church at the time — it was a Sunday evening — and she grabbed my neck and squeezed me so hard that I nearly wrecked the car.

❧

The decision to get married was the third big decision I had made in less than two years, and one that would, like the first, have an incalculable impact on my life. (I'm not sure about the decision to go to Baylor, although it doubtless had an important effect as well.) Logically speaking, Anne and I were too young to consider marriage. Anne was only sixteen and I was eighteen. But we had both learned a lot of responsibility early in life, and, more importantly, we loved each other too much to wait.

At first we intended to delay marrying until I finished college. But when Anne's father said he would send her to college only if she went to one I wasn't attending, she said, "Let's go ahead and get married and I'll work until you graduate."

So we set the date for the following June, on my nineteenth birthday. Anne, who was seventeen, had just finished high school. We found a small apartment for thirty-five dollars a month, which we painted, decorated, and outfitted with cast-off furniture. And we still managed, out of my twenty-five-dollar-a-week salary, to save a hundred dollars that summer. At the end of the summer, with the money in hand, we set out in a 1939 Ford for Waco, Texas, so I could complete my work at Baylor.

Our old car, which was a wedding present from my parents, burned a quart of oil every hundred miles. I bought a whole case of cheap motor oil — I think it cost six dollars for twenty-four quarts — and stopped beside the road every hundred miles to add a quart to the engine.

While I was at Georgetown College I had taken several correspondence courses at Baylor. So by taking a heavy class load I was able to complete my undergraduate work at Baylor in a single year. I worked part-time in a bookstore. Anne found employment as a secretary in a local drug company, earning the grand sum of thirty dollars a week. We were almost desperately poor, but we were so happy to be together that we didn't notice.

֍

Eventually Anne earned more than the equivalent of a university degree, taking courses at the University of Kentucky, George Peabody College for Teachers, and the New England Conservatory of Music. She taught piano for two years at Georgetown College in Kentucky and later at a parochial school in Nashville, Tennessee. She composed several musicals and a number of hymns, and published two novels and a book of meditations. For eight years she was the organist of the Little Stone Church on Mackinac Island, Michigan, where visitors often commented on how spellbinding the music was.

I often reflect on what a wonderful woman she is, and how lucky I was, understanding as little about human personality and potential as I did, to marry a girl like her. In addition to being one of the most creative and imaginative homemakers in the world, and to being the most consistently exciting and caring mother our two sons could have had, she has been a beautiful, resourceful, and completely satisfying mate, always bringing far more to our relationship than I'm afraid I was able to bring.

Anne is one of the truly exceptional people I have known in my lifetime, and, while I think she always worried that I might find another woman more attractive, I have to confess that I never did. She has been a dream of a partner for more than half a century!

֍

When we left Waco I was still only nineteen and didn't feel mature enough to go to seminary. So we returned to Kentucky, where the people at another church had been asking about the possibility of my becoming their pastor. It was called Poplar Grove Baptist Church because it sat in a little grove of tall poplar trees in rural Rockcastle County, "twenty miles, two hoots, and a holler," as they said, from any kind of civilization. Only two members of the congregation had ever been to college, but the people were all eager to support a young pastor and his wife who wanted to go to school.

So I became their minister and enrolled in a master's program in English at the University of Kentucky. The chemistry was great, both at the church and at the university. I felt so enriched by my year earning a master's degree that I decided to stay and attempt a doctorate as well. And I was learning almost as much from my simple parishioners, albeit in a different vein, as I was from my erudite professors at the university. It was an incredibly rich and satisfying life!

Then came another momentous decision: where to go to seminary.

I had never questioned where I would attend seminary. I assumed it would be at Southern Baptist Theological Seminary in Louisville, the most prestigious of six large seminaries operated by Southern Baptists. But when I drove up to the seminary to talk about getting a church closer to Louisville (because I could no longer afford to drive the greater distance to the little parish I had) the dean was cavalier to the point of being rude. He told me that I would simply have to have enough faith to come and wait for the Lord to provide another situation.

Disappointed, I returned home to find a letter from Harvard Divinity School offering me a full fellowship and an additional stipend. The stipend wasn't large, but it didn't take me long to make up my mind. In August 1957, after a summer when I worked as a salesman in a Baker's Qualicraft Shoe Store and Anne was the secretary of the Kentucky Medical Foundation, we packed our belongings in our car — this time a 1949 Chrysler — and headed for Cambridge, Massachusetts.

Reflecting on that move, Anne and I agree that it was one of the most important we ever made, for it cast us immediately into an environment as foreign as if we had traveled to China or South America. Sometimes we could barely understand the New England accent, with its nasality, its broad *a*'s, and its frequent addition of unwarranted *r*'s at the end of words ending in vowels. After I made some friends there, I teased them about saying "Fath*a*h is sitting on the sof*er*." (The first *a* is short, like the *a* in "had.") Shortly after we arrived on the Harvard campus, I was asked by a visitor if I could direct him to the *PEEB'idy MUS'*ium. He repeated it several times, each time very quickly, before I finally realized that he was asking for what I, as a Southerner, would have called the Pea*BOD'y MuSE'*um.

We were fortunate, shortly after arriving in Cambridge, to receive a call to a small church in North Reading, Massachusetts, just south of Andover, that had a delightful, relatively new Cape Cod parsonage. I say we were fortunate, because otherwise, even with my stipend from Harvard, it would have been financially impossible for us to remain in that very expensive area. In six weeks we had almost exhausted the thousand dollars we had managed to save before leaving Kentucky.

It was an exceptionally good time to be at Harvard Divinity School. Paul Tillich, the famous existentialist theologian, was working out his *Systematic Theology* there as well as teaching courses in the Reformation, and George Huntston Williams was giving his masterful lectures on church history. Paul Lehman was painstakingly completing his *chef d'oeuvre* on Christian ethics. Robert Pfeiffer, the brilliant Old Testament scholar, died after my first year, but was replaced by G. Ernest Wright and Frank Cross Jr., two of the most articulate younger scholars in the field, who were intimately involved in the translation and interpretation of the recently discovered Dead Sea Scrolls. Amos Wilder and Krister Stendahl, very different New Testament scholars, one already world-famous and the other fast becoming so, shared the task of initiating us into the mystery of the Gospels and Pauline epistles.

Two other men, both ministers, had an enormous influence on me. One was Samuel H. Miller, who was still pastor of the Old Cambridge Baptist Church when I took his course in theology and literature (he would later become dean of the Harvard Divinity School). The other was George A. Buttrick, the idiosyncratic but extremely effective Preacher to the University (the official title for the university chaplain) and the Divinity School's professor of homiletics and church administration.

Buttrick would play an important role in my life, not only for his lectures in the classroom and example in the pulpit, but also because he would, a few years later when I had gone on to take a doctorate at Princeton and then become dean of a liberal arts college in Louisville, recommend my appointment to the faculty at Vanderbilt Divinity School in Nashville, thus rescuing me from administrative work (I was beginning to get offers of college presidencies) and setting me up for fifteen years of the most creative and exciting work I would ever do.

There was not much decision involved in making that move. I did not like being an administrator. I was a reasonably good one, I think, and some of the professors I hired generously credited me later with the inspiration to become superb administrators themselves. But as I have sometimes characterized the job of being a dean, it means minding everybody's business but your own. I wanted to think and write and speak, not organize curricula, interview potential faculty members, listen to complaints, and preside over an endless stream of committee meetings.

So the opportunity to escape to a teaching job at Vanderbilt, even though it meant an enormous reduction in salary, didn't raise a whisper of a question in my mind. Nor would I ever question it later. It was precisely the situation I needed in which to discover the limits of my talents, the direction of my mind and heart, and the joys of being a husband and father.

☙

Looking back now, I can only shake my head in wonder at how crucial those early choices were for the way my life and thought have developed. Did I really make the choices or were they made for me? Did I actually face them for the dramatic forks in the road I now realize they were, or did some beneficent higher power set them up so that I couldn't bungle them, the way George Plimpton said the "paper tigers" of American industry are provided with prearranged choices in which they can seldom err?

Perhaps it was similar ruminations that caused the Apostle Paul, in his Letter to the Romans, to get into the matter of predestination, and try to explain how we could be both foreordained and free in the mind of God. I made the decisions, yet they were in some mysterious way made before I made them, and had an inherent inevitability about them that I could not overrule.

The choices I did make, or accept after they were made for me, seem so indivisibly a part of my existence, so inseparable from who I was and am and shall be, that they are the stuff of my very soul. I would not be who I am apart from them. Therefore I marvel at them and celebrate them, and in some way celebrate life and God for them.

Every biography is a model of this miraculous development. We make crucial decisions along the way, but we still have to marvel at the way our lives unfolded, at the manifold circumstances that always dictated the choices we were offered, at the concatenation of people and events that guided us from the point where we joined the road to the point where we look back and say, "That was an amazing journey!"

☙

For me, there were still other important choices to come, although, occurring further along life's way, they could not begin to compare with the earlier ones for the depth and breadth of their impact. One was to leave the comparatively safe, comfortable environment of the university to become the minister of a congregation again. Another, several years later, was to leave the now-familiar, intoxicating world of the large church to return to a professorate. And still another was to turn my back on the professorate and semiretire, spending my summers on Mackinac Island, Michigan, as minister of a small resort church and having the rest of the year free to write, travel, and explore new pathways of the soul.

But before any of these choices there came a very important one about the nature of life and thought. It occurred in the midst of a wonderful year we spent living in Paris, France. When I went to Vanderbilt Divinity School as a young professor, there was a rotation plan in the faculty for sending members away on sabbatical leave. The preaching department, which I shared with a fine, elderly gentleman named John Irwin, was due for one of its members to go on sabbatical in 1967–68, my third year at the university. John didn't want to go. He was too old, he said, and he and his wife didn't need the stress of relocation at their time of life. So by default the privilege fell to me.

What should I do with the opportunity? A couple of years earlier, when I was teaching courses in theology and literature at the University of Chicago for Professor Nathan A. Scott Jr., while he was on leave, I had become quite interested in the theater of the absurd, and felt that there were febrile relationships between the exciting drama of experimentalists such as Samuel Beckett and Eugene Ionesco and the cultural change I could sense occurring in theology and the church. So I drafted a proposal to go to France and study the theater of the absurd at its historical and spiritual center, with the idea of producing a book about the interrelationship of the new theater and the new theology. The proposal was approved by the university research council and, even better, won generous financial support from the American Council of Learned Societies and the American Association of Theological Schools. We were going to Europe on an income twice as large as the one I had been earning at the university! The experience changed our lives completely — or at least confirmed changes that were already occurring without our notice.

The year in Paris was virtually indescribable for its magic and joy. I served as theologian-in-residence at the American Church in Paris, a beautiful edifice on the Left Bank of the Seine not far from the Eiffel Tower. This provided us with a garret apartment on the fourth floor of the church building, from whose windows we had marvelous views of the Seine and the famous rooftops of Paris across the river. Each day we shopped for our food in the little stalls two or three blocks behind the church, and learned to converse in halting French with the smiling, friendly shop-keepers. Our sons attended a British school on the other side of the river, the path to which led us over the Pont d'Alma and past the Crazy Horse Saloon, whose door was always guarded by a large man in the colorful uniform of a Canadian Mountie. I taught a Sunday school class — the only adult class — in the church each week, and met dozens of American businessmen and their wives who have remained our friends ever since. We also got to know a couple of French families extremely well and spent many happy hours with them.

In my research into the subject of absurd drama I tried to visit as many productions of the absurdists' works as possible, and this led inadvertently to one of the most profound spiritual experiences of my life. I had gone on a bright Sunday afternoon in April to the little Théâtre du Rochechouart on a quiet back street of Paris to see a performance of Spanish playwright Fernando Arrabal's *Le Cimetière des voitures (The Car Cemetery)*. It was a tiny theater and the stage had been constructed around all four walls of the room, with stairs that permitted the audience to climb up and over into the center as we entered. Once we were inside and the performance began, however, the stairs were removed, leaving us virtual captives in our arena of swiveling seats.

The director of the play was a disciple of Antonin Artaud, the fa-mous dadaist, whose book *The Theater and Its Double* proposed that plays should assume an almost militaristic, interrogational posture toward the audience, assaulting it with lights, noise, and even insults. Accordingly the performance was highly cacophonous, with the actors continuously yelling, stomping around, and using pieces of tailpipe to bang on the hulks of old cars and sheets of metal hanging around the stage. Numerous klieg lights rotated constantly, nearly blinding us as they did.

I thought I would go mad in the first five minutes! Only a punk-rocker accustomed to blaring amplifiers and the strobing glare of revolving lamps could have been comfortable in such an antagonistic environment.

But there was no way out. The stairs had been removed and the doors were shut. We were there for the duration.

I don't know how long it took — perhaps half an hour — but eventually I became inured to the madness of the performance and began to follow it with interest, turning this way and that toward the various stages. By the time the play was over I had not only come to appreciate it but, in some odd, unexplainable way, even to enjoy it.

Accordingly, when the play ended, the stairs were restored, and we tumbled out blindly into the late afternoon sunshine, I felt very strange. Everything was so quiet. I could hear a dog barking in the distance, and children playing somewhere. But that was all. It is hard to describe what I actually felt, but it was accompanied by a strong suspicion that the world into which I had now stepped was unreal, while the world inside the theater was the real one. I suddenly wanted to turn back and reenter the world from which I had just emerged.

This was probably the second-most-important experience of my life. The first, I believe, was the day I became a Christian, and assumed the lifelong journey of a follower of Jesus. More than anything else, that conversion has affected everything about my existence. But the second experience was to determine a great deal of how I would act out the first experience, for it reminded me, in the most forceful way, that reality is largely a matter of the environment in which we come to understand it. In psychological terms, reality is "socially constructed." That is, each of us perceives it in terms of how it is interpreted by our most immediate society — our families, our friends, and our communities.

It would be difficult to overestimate the significance of such a discovery. I had grown up in a small town in Kentucky and much of my worldview was shaped by the Southern Baptist church to which I belonged. I had believed, because it was what I was taught, that God created the world in six days, God sent Jesus into the world to die for people's sins, people were going to hell if they didn't accept the sacrificial death of Christ in their behalf, and the best thing anybody could do in return for God's mercy was to become a preacher and tell others about it. Now, years after I had been to Harvard and Princeton, I saw with a clarity I had never experienced that the "truth" one believes is largely conditioned by the culture in which one grew up. Our worldviews and attitudes toward life are almost entirely formed by the important people in our lives — parents, friends, teachers, and heroes — and most of us never go beyond these views and attitudes or surrender them for others that might possibly be more faithful to reality.

Maybe other people realized this much earlier than I did, and I was only slow to come to it. But to me it was an earthshaking idea, one that would set me on the road to enormous mutations of thought and energy!

I can only wonder now how I would have reacted to Jerry Falwell when I moved to Lynchburg, Virginia, if I had not had that experience in Paris. Perhaps I would have accepted Falwell's vision of life and the world as being only a fundamentalist version of the one I held growing up, and would not have spoken out against it. I doubt if I would have seen so clearly the things I eventually pilloried in *Ten Things I Learned Wrong from a Conservative Church*. Nor would I attempt to write the book I am now planning to write, *God by Any Other Name: The Deity of the Coming Global Religion*. My whole understanding of religion, and my commitment to following Christ, was vastly altered by that single insight from a tiny theater on the back streets of Paris.

⁓

Talk about the importance of choices! There are choices we all make that establish a series of consequences for the remainder of our lives. Where we go to school, who we marry, how we enter the work force, and dozens of other decisions continue to exert an influence on us until the day we die — and perhaps, if we believe in the afterlife, even beyond death.

Wrong choices are just as important in our lives as right ones. In fact, it is often difficult to determine which choices were wrong and which were right. I sometimes ask what would have happened to me if I had not married the wonderful woman I married, or had not decided to become a minister, or had not gone to the schools I went to, or had not had one foot in the academic world and another in the church, or had not forsaken the Southern Baptists to become a Presbyterian and later a Congregationalist.

In the end, I think, we should not spend our time mourning the things that did not come about in our lives, but should instead give thanks for the experiences we did have and the persons we did know and love. People who are constantly bemoaning the decisions they made and the paths their lives have taken are obviously not at peace with themselves. They are unable to step back from their existences and say, "I've had a lovely life and God has been very good to me. I am grateful for the journey I have made, and would not have it any other way."

For my part, I am glad to bless God for the paths I have taken. I cannot help wondering sometimes what would have happened if I had done this or that — if I had become an artist, if I had taken a church in New York City, if I had stayed in my job at Vanderbilt University. It is natural to speculate. But it is important to be grateful for everything that happened just as it happened, and not to be always wishing things were different. John Cage, the famous musicologist, had the right idea when he said, "Everything is music, and everywhere is the best seat."

Everywhere *is* the best seat. Every life is beautiful. Life itself is beautiful. It is important to know this and to accept it in the deepest parts of our psyches. Then we can join the ancient psalmist in exclaiming,

> Bless the Lord, O my soul,
> and all that is within me,
> bless his holy name.
>
> (Psalm 103:1)

Three

For the Fun of It!

One of my favorite things is to remember the good times I have had. I play them again and again in my mind, like favorite recordings, and each time they bless my life all over again. My wife says I have a facility for forgetting the bad times and remembering only the good ones. That isn't really true. I am able to recall the bad times too. But I think I have a little mechanism inside that doesn't let me play those as often as I play the good things. And as I grow older I really want to play those good times as much as possible. There seems to be a kind of health and joy in doing so.

Despite the fact that my home wasn't always happy because my father continually threatened to break it up, I recall many wonderful moments from my childhood. A lot of these moments centered on Christmas. My dad was often childlike then, and we saw a side of him we seldom saw at other times. He loved the presents, the lights, the color, the foods and smells of Christmas, and often wrote us little notes from Santa after consuming the milk and cookies we had left for him.

Many of my favorite gifts in those years came from my aunt in Iowa. Aunt Lulu was a large, jovial German woman who never married but stayed on the farm to care for my grandparents until they died. Even though she never had children of her own, she had a knack for selecting presents children would like — colorful, unique things, such as a mechanical dog that barked and turned flips and a little car that bumped into things and changed direction when it did. Clearly, Aunt Lulu remembered the joy of play and shared that joy with me.

My solitary play activities in those days centered on two places. One was a large wooden packing crate in what we called the "junk room" of the house, where I crawled in with my toys and played when the weather was cold or inclement. The other was the hollow area under a large spirea bush that grew next to our house. The bush rose like a fountain and sent its branches into great splashing arcs, providing a generous play space and lots of privacy beneath them. I loved playing under that bush because it was my secret domain.

From my earliest years I had a special fondness for the outdoors and loved to explore woods and fields and creeks. My father usually planted some kind of winter crop on our garden, winter wheat or crimson clover, both of which grew tall and thick, and I delighted in getting down and crawling through the overgrowth, imagining that I was invisible to the world.

Later, when my father's work took us to Somerset, Kentucky, and he bought a small farm on the edge of town, I spent hours almost every day roaming up and down a small creek or just sitting among the rocks on a steep hillside. When I began to become religious and learned to pray, this area became my leafy temple, where I felt closer to God than anywhere else in the world.

I wasn't really a recluse, though. I also joined in seasonal games — football, basketball, baseball — with the neighborhood children. Our basketball court consisted of a narrow strip of land between a tobacco field and an old barn, where the rusty metal rim of a lard can nailed to the barn served as a hoop. Our football games were played on a field where a farmer raised corn in the spring and summer, and when we began playing in the fall we had to be careful of the short, ragged stalks left standing after the corn was harvested. There would be eight or ten of us neighborhood boys in the game, four or five on each side. I almost always played quarterback. Even now, more than half a century later, I can easily recall the thrill of running, dodging, throwing the football, and making touchdowns.

On summer evenings, we played a lot of hide-and-seek. As many as a dozen children would flee from the person who was "it," like phantoms disappearing into the shadows, and it often took half an hour to turn up all the missing players. One of the memories I have of this is the time I crawled onto the corrugated-tin roof of an outbuilding to hide and found the younger sister of one of my friends already hiding there. We lay there side by side for several minutes while the person who was "it" searched for us. It was a very hot, sticky evening, and the girl, a sultry thirteen-year-old who looked like a pretty, full-bodied gypsy, appeared very warm and clammy in the last rays of the sun. For the first time since I had known her, I realized she was turning into a desirable young woman.

I still remember the spent-but-happy feeling I had when play was over and it was time to go home and get cleaned up for bed. There was something enormously satisfying about the way full play used up my supply of energy and left me with a smile in my heart. I was tired but I was also immensely satisfied, as if I had performed the way a child should perform at that age and was at peace with the world.

༄

Several years later, I would read Johan Huizinga's classic volume *Homo Ludens,* or *Man at Play.* Huizinga, a Dutch sociologist, believed that people are never more authentically themselves than when they are playing. Much of what is wrong with the adult world, he said, is that people get involved in their routine existence and no longer play, or, what is worse, even forget how to play.

Shortly after my discovery of Huizenga several books on so-called "play theology" appeared, including Sam Keen's *To a Dancing God,* Robert Neale's *In Praise of Play,* Harvey Cox's *A Feast of Fools,* and Jürgen Moltmann's *A Theology of Play.* The general thesis of these books was that human beings are much more natural when they are playing than when they are working. They are also more capable of real spirituality when they are playing, for then they are in a more natural state with God.

Fascinated by the implications of these ideas for worship, I wrote a book called *Leave It to the Spirit: Commitment and Freedom in the New Liturgy*, in which I made a pitch for more play and imagination in the way we worship God in our churches. Most worship services were such staid and routine affairs, I argued, that they failed to offer full involvement to the minds, hearts, and bodies of the participants, and thus fell short of the ideal of true worship, that it should actually involve worshipers in acts of renewal and recreation. This criticism was particularly true with regard to the body, which had become anathema to most churches in the Reformed tradition, where thinking God's thoughts after him was much preferred to mimicking any kind of divine actions. It is important, I said, to reclaim the use of the body in worship, and to learn to move with the kind of freedom exemplified in Pentecostal or African-American worship. In other words, I was advising the return to play or full involvement, not just mental activity, in Protestant worship.

At the time, I was teaching a seminar in experimental preaching at Vanderbilt Divinity School, trying to loosen up the students and help them to go beyond older, more sanctified styles of preaching to more novel and imaginative forms. Participants in the seminar created many fascinating homilies using various musical, theatrical, and media forms. Some of these were so excitingly innovative that I gathered them into two published volumes, *Experimental Preaching* and *The Eleven O'Clock News & Other Experimental Sermons*. As a prelude to each seminar, I assigned members to prepare play-and-relaxation exercises for us to do as a group. One married couple in the seminar designed an exercise using body painting. I'll never forget the sight of one fifty-five-year-old minister, pastor of a prominent local Presbyterian church, lying shirtless on a pad, his pant legs rolled up to his knees, while half a dozen students finger-painted colorful designs on his pale legs and torso. At first, he was nervous, but then he began to giggle at the squishy feeling of the fingers applying the paint. Afterward he confessed to me that that session literally changed his life and gave him a totally different attitude toward himself and his work.

I was clearly on pilgrimage during those years toward a more liberated experience of my own. Always work-oriented, I had earned two academic doctorates, written many books and articles, and pushed myself to answer speaking invitations from around the country. Now, in midlife, I was feeling the need to reclaim the playful aspect of my self, to integrate my self as a whole being capable of living, thinking, and existing imaginatively, above the humdrum necessities imposed by the workaday world. And it was out of this wholeness, eventually, that I responded to a call to forsake the safe, tenured realm of the university and become a full-time minister in a busy, high-pressure church.

One of the things I insisted on when I accepted the invitation of the First Presbyterian Church of Lynchburg, Virginia, to come as their pastor was a generous amount of time off for recreating myself and rethinking my way on a continual basis. The church normally gave its ministers a four-week annual vacation and a two-week study leave. I asked for ten weeks in all, defined any way they would like, and got them, reminding the negotiators that this was not an unusual request in light of the tradition among New York ministers who received entire summers away. I did the same when I left Lynchburg and went to the First Congregational Church of Los Angeles. The reason I was being called to those churches, I argued, was that I was a creative, highly responsible minister. If they wished me to remain that way then I must have the time to read, think, play, and create.

Looking back, I believe this arrangement was one of the most important factors of my ministries in those churches. The crucial thing, I always felt, was to retain my sense of playfulness, my ability to immerse myself in nonprofessional activities and feel vitally refreshed and reinvigorated. It is so easy, when one is at the mercy of a harrowing schedule most of the time, to lose oneself in a forest of activities where there are few clearings and the undergrowth soon becomes suffocating.

∾

I have always loved a chapter title in Dom Aelred Graham's book *Zen Catholicism*. He called it "The Importance of Not Being Earnest." The chapter was about Catholicism's need for the playful spirit of Zen Buddhism, so that it can rise above its dogmatic, practical approach to everything. There is a subtlety and complexity in the phrase, to be sure. It means more than merely abandoning our sensible pursuits in favor of having fun. It means — well, not taking ourselves so damned seriously.

I have often found it true that I needed to transcend my own seriousness — even to take a hike from my practical, pragmatic side and engage in risky thought or behavior. This is where the spirit of playfulness comes in. It permits us to transcend our usual, workaday estimates of life and the way things are, and to abandon ourselves, at least occasionally, to impractical roles and directions in our lives.

The secret of play is to become so caught up in what one is doing that for a little while at least the rest of the world ceases to exist. Time flies and everything else is forgotten. What one is presently playing at has become the most important thing in one's existence.

Several years ago I had a remarkable dream that characterizes my enthusiasm for playing. The dream occurred in three consecutive installments with brief intervals between them. In the first part, I was a turtle paddling slowly about in some algae-rich primeval pool, my eyes slightly above the water level, luxuriating in the nascency of everything. In the second part, I was a medieval monk in a monastery, contentedly copying a manuscript. And, in the third installment, I was Genghis Khan, riding through enemy hordes at full throttle, striking in every direction with my flashing scimitar.

When I told the dream to my wife, Anne, she exclaimed, "Why, you're all three of those!"

She was right. The dream had exquisitely captured the most important facets of my personality. Like the turtle, I enjoy being an observer in a world still coming into being, and am never more content than when I am lazily swimming along with my eyes just above the surface of the water. Like the monk, I spend a great deal of my time scribbling, and treasure a quiet, meditative environment in which to do it. And like Genghis Khan, I ride boldly into almost everything I do, swinging right and left as if my life depended on it.

The thing about real play is that it is so absorbing — that one truly pours oneself into it with such total abandon that for a while it becomes one's world, one's only reality. The absorption factor is one of the gauges by which we know if we are engaged in play and not in some facsimile of it.

I always liked the little Zen story about the monk Ryokan. He loved to play with children and did so with such intensity that one night when he was playing hide-and-seek with them and their mothers called them to dinner, he remained all night in the haystack where he was hiding. When the farmer came the next morning to get some hay for his cattle, Ryokan motioned him to silence, lest the children hear.

There is something godlike about such fierce involvement, I think — something admirable and transcendent, especially when the player is an adult. It ignores all the constructs of the outer world and treats the play world as a supreme reality.

∽

At some deep, unconscious level we are aware of a strong element of play in the universe itself — of a playfulness so vital and meaningful to everything that God too is involved in it. This is one reason primitive religions all depended on mimetic action to get God to do things: rain dances to invoke rain for crops, imitation hunts to summon divine aid in killing wild animals, and healing rituals to invite God's resuscitation of sick or dying individuals.

When we play, therefore, we are either consciously or unconsciously participating in this transcendent dimension of life. There is something that feels right and good about real play, whether it is in a ball game, on a golf course, at the card table, on the dance floor, or in some enormous practical joke. We feel truly alive when we are playing, probably more alive than at any other time.

For some of us — and I admit that I am one — even work can be play. When we are absorbed by what we are doing, whether it is planting a garden, making a piece of furniture, designing a new computer program, or writing a book, we aren't aware that we are working. On the contrary, we are so totally involved that we feel reinvigorated by what we are doing. We become fully alive while we are caught up in whatever it is we are working on.

Somehow, at a level of spiritual cosmology we seldom contemplate, being at play means participating in the created order the way we were intended to be involved with it. Then we are like NFL players who demonstrate who they really are by getting off the bench and becoming totally absorbed in the game on the field. It is that for which we exist. This is why we say of people who never play, who keep their noses to the grindstone and refuse to disport themselves, that they haven't lived. In a sense, they haven't. They are like Ebenezer Scrooge in his counting house, denying the higher and better instincts of their lives. We applaud when the three ghosts finally shake Scrooge out of his lethargy and involve him once more in life. It is a transcendent moment in Dickens's beautiful story. But it is the moment we are all meant to have, the conversion we are all intended to undergo. This, I believe, is the reason for the incredible, continuing success of *A Christmas Carol;* it is a dramatization of the action to which we are all meant to succumb, an action which in religious terms is tantamount to salvation.

ↄ

Most playing is obviously more suited to people in their retirement period than in their harder time of struggling to survive and provide something in reserve for their later years. There is a release that comes with retirement, a gratifying sense that it is now time for play and relaxation. We naturally smile at bumper stickers on older couples' RVs that say, "We are spending our children's inheritance." Good for them, we think — they have earned this time of happiness and exploration! Retired people often speak of having discovered their "second childhood" — of learning to frolic and play all over again.

The movie *Cocoon,* starring Jessica Tandy and Don Ameche, is a classic example of this. *Cocoon* is the story of a group of elderly people in Florida who are mysteriously rejuvenated by a radioactive object they encounter on a fishing trip. Their contact with the object transforms them into youths again without altering their appearance. Soon they are amazing everybody by playing smash volleyball, dancing with abandon, swimming and diving, and generally cavorting like children instead of the elder adults they appear to be. The thing that touches the hearts of this film's viewing audience, I think, is the appropriateness of the characters' being able to play again. In a perfect world — perhaps in the next one? — people enjoy both the wisdom of age and the playfulness of youth.

❧

Travel is another way many of us play, particularly travel that is adventurous. I have always found that being in exotic or unfamiliar settings has been an enormous stimulus to my sensibilities, enabling me to escape my ordinary frame of reference. I often think of Franz Kafka's love of strange cities. He said there is a kind of eroticism about them, an appeal that goes to the very heart and soul of who we are.

I remember, when Anne and I had been married four years, our first trip to Florida. We had very little money, so we rented a tiny, self-catering cabin at Indian Rocks Beach, near St. Petersburg, where Anne prepared all our food. But the tropical setting — palm trees rustling in the breeze, blistering temperatures (it was July!), and some of the most colorful sunsets we had ever seen — was so different for us that it was like being in a foreign country.

So was our life in New England, where I attended Harvard Divinity School and Anne went to the New England Conservatory of Music. Our little parsonage there sat on a hill above a small lake called Martin's Pond. In the fall we viewed with amazement the glorious colors of the great oak and maple trees, and spent our spare moments around Concord and Lexington, where the trees appeared brightest and loveliest. In winter, when the lake was frozen, we went ice skating. In spring and summer there were the ocean and all the little seaports with gulls screaming overhead. Our favorite places were Rockport and Marblehead. We would buy a loaf of fresh bread, a slab of cheese, some apples, and a bottle of sauterne, and go out among the rocks at the Marblehead lighthouse, where we watched the sailboats skimming in and out like moths cruising around an old wool sweater.

Our next huge adventure was the year we went on sabbatical to England and Paris. We sailed on the SS *France* for Southampton, where we had a little red Volkswagen Squareback waiting, and drove through tree-shaded lanes into the West End of London. For six weeks we "did" all the sights in London and its suburbs, reveling in the city of Shakespeare and Christopher Wren, James Boswell and Samuel Johnson, Charles Dickens and T. S. Eliot. One day we visited Thomas Carlyle's house in Cheney Row, where the doughty old Scotsman had received the great composer Chopin. When the docent learned that Anne was a pianist, he invited her to sit and play at the spinet piano Chopin had used when he was there. It was a magical moment for both of us!

After London we motored up through Cambridge and York to Edinburgh and eventually as far as Inverness. On our way back south, we discovered the incredible beauty of the English Lake District, where Wordsworth and Southey had lived, and saw one of Shakespeare's plays at

Stratford, his hometown on the river Avon. For someone who had taken a doctorate in English literature, this was a dream come true.

On the continent, we experienced the same kind of euphoria — dancing among the late-evening shadows of the Black Forest, wandering the back streets of Paris, marveling at the ancient blue and red glass in the cathedral at Chartres, kissing in the moonlight on Mont St. Michel, sipping Cokes at sidewalk cafés in Segovia, shopping on the Ponte Vecchio in Florence, eating cheese fondue with the yodelers in a tavern in Lucerne, cooling our feet in the sea at Bibbona.

In succeeding years, our travels would take us all over the globe — to Greece, Israel, Hong Kong, Japan, Thailand, the Philippines, even Vietnam while Seoul was being shelled. When our oldest son Eric graduated from high school, he and I took a walking trip through the Greek Isles, riding ferries and cattle-boats from island to island, then backpacking across the islands and catching boats from the other side.

As I look back on those days, I realize how truly playful — i.e., full of play — they were, how carefree and engrossing and liberating. We were often so absorbed in what we were seeing and doing that there was a kind of unawareness of self, a submersion of self in a sea of enormous joy.

It is hard to imagine that one soul is the repository of so many grand memories. It is an understatement to say that travel broadens, for it does much more than that. Like play — for that is what travel at its best is — it fills the heart with shining experiences. And just as play expands the boundaries of our lives and imagination, so does travel. It reminds us of how limited our own country and background are beside the myriads of cultures and experiences in other parts of the world. It conditions us to believe that heaven will have to be very exceptional — in a word, it must be *heaven!* — in order not to pale beside the beauties and extravagances of this present world.

ᴄ⋄

I have been talking about how the fun or play of my life — the things that have brought me joy and diversion and excitement — contributes to my sense of spirituality in my elder years. The memories of those things still excite me, still make me feel the wonder and electricity I felt then. These are part of my soul, part of my very being in God. I can only be grateful for them, and, in thanking God, feel more accepted by God, more intimate with God.

The thing is, they remind me that life is always much bigger and deeper than I can ever imagine.

The Latin word *ludere*, "to play," has many meanings — to frolic and gambol, as a child or a puppy does; to enact on a stage, thereby creating an illusion of something; to pretend, thus establishing a situation or a world different from the one around us; to rearrange things in order to impart a different meaning for them or to call attention to a particular segment of them; to imitate an action, either divine or human, and thus to give it a new extension in reality.

When we play at anything it means that we enter an aspect of reality *as if* it were reality itself, thereby bestowing on that aspect a kind of reality that cannot always be detected from more basic reality. We enter a new state of mind with such intensity that, for a little while at least, that state of mind consciously or unconsciously becomes our reality. Of course it doesn't necessarily make that reality *the* reality, for *the* reality is usually waiting for us when the illusion of that one fades or ceases to be. The house is still a mess when we return from the ball, there are still the tax returns to finish when we go home from the movie, we are still wearing braces after fantasizing we were kissing a movie star. Yet in some mysterious way *that* reality participates in *the* reality, and vice versa. For all reality is of a piece, even the parts of it that we only fancy or imagine. It is all a part of life, of *our* lives, and, as such, affects everything that is. And it is all part of living before God.

I am acutely conscious of this as I grow older and am learning to cele-brate it as part of my spirituality. I can't explain it, and confess that I don't fully understand it. Yet it is inseparable from the mystery of the life that is lived in the presence of God. I am not even sure I want to understand it; to do so might rob it of some of its beauty and allure. I am only a creature — one who has, to be sure, struggled to comprehend the world and my relationship to it. But in the end my very creatureliness means that I can't understand, that I am destined, at best, to acknowledge my unworthiness and to fall down and worship the God who presides over everything.

Is there no delight in this? On the contrary, there is enormous delight! I can't believe that I would be half so happy if I were able to grasp everything perfectly, for then I would stand in the isolation of my own achievement instead of having this crazy, warm, fuzzy feeling that I am accepted by God as part of the glorious mystery simply *because* I am so imperfect and can't begin to grasp it. Doesn't that make sense, at least religiously? I revel in the fact that the multiple realities of life whirl around me like the lights from a mirror-ball twirling on the ceiling of a dance hall, for I believe that in the final analysis Calvin was right, "Man's chief end is to worship God and enjoy Him forever."

This is precisely what I have been talking about!

Four

Life Is What You Read into It

Comic books were my first serious reading. My father was never much of a reader. *His* most serious reading was agricultural reports and *Popular Mechanics.* But for some reason he was greatly enamored of the comic books that began appearing when I was about four or five, and used to bring home a couple of new ones every Friday evening. He read them first, and when he finished he gave them to me. My favorites were Superman, Batman and Robin, Captain Marvel, and Spider-Man. I liked Wonder Woman too, but always had the feeling that she was inferior to the others. That must have been an incipient anti-feminism.

I wish I had saved the early editions of those comic books. Today they would be worth a fortune. I read each of them several times, then traded or sold them to other children in the neighborhood. At Christmas I usually wrapped up several and gave them to classmates, especially poorer boys I figured never got any on their own.

I had learned to read by watching the words as my mother read to me and my little sister. I was three the Christmas she sat down to read us *The Night Before Christmas* and I surprised her by reading it aloud. So I was ready to read the comic books when Dad started buying them. I think it was from them, more than Sunday school and the Bible, that I first learned my lifelong lessons about honesty, justice, and the proper use of force. I continued to like them for years.

I read the obligatory childhood books too — the Hardy boys, Booth Tarkington, *Huckleberry Finn* and *Tom Sawyer*, *Black Beauty*, Robert Louis Stevenson's *A Child's Garden of Verses*, and a few other classics. But none of them with the passion I felt for a good comic book.

In my teen years I began to read the Bible religiously, and in this case I think the pun makes sense. I was reading it for the meaning of life. I regarded it as a very sacred book — too sacred ever to mark in. And I often memorized little verses that meant a lot to me, so that as an adult I can quote long passages of scripture from memory, although the many versions I have read now tend to become confused in my mind and I can't always get the phrasing precisely right.

For me personally, the most influential writer I read in high school was probably Ralph Waldo Emerson. His essay "Self-Reliance" really enthralled me. Already I was hungering for some validation of my sense of independence, and when I read things such as "Trust thyself; every heart vibrates to that iron string," and "Whoso would be a man, must be a non-conformist," my spirit resonated with them like a tuning fork. The complete volume of Emerson's essays was one of the first books I ever purchased. It was in the old Modern Library edition and cost a dollar-twenty-five. I still have it, and enjoy turning the pages and seeing the passages I marked as a teenager.

Now, years later, I realize how much Emerson's sonorous statements did to shape my philosophy, and possibly to form my diction as well. In 2003, on the two-hundredth anniversary of the Sage of Concord's birth, I reread most of his essays and found them amazingly prescient. I built a sermon around some of them. With only minor adaptations, they would still sound wonderfully fresh and commanding in the lecture hall today.

In college, it was the British romantic poets who attracted me most — particularly Wordsworth, with his psalming of nature and the God of wild places. I was into nature myself then, having spent a lot of time in the woods. Later I would enjoy Thoreau's *Walden Pond,* and feel when I actually visited Walden that I was walking through sacred groves. But before

Thoreau it was Wordsworth who took me by the hand and taught me what my heart was feeling.

It was in reading Wordsworth that I first truly understood the biblical psalms, and what the psalmists were trying to express. The psalms were not literal truth and were certainly not meant to be read literally. They were poetic renditions of outbursts of feeling, of emotions welling up from the depths of the soul and seeking crystallization in words as a way of preserving the emotions themselves. When the twenty-third Psalm says, "Yea, though I walk through the valley of the shadow of death," we are suddenly there, treading that awful valley, feeling the oppressive weight of some great loss or affliction, and finding hope in the affirmation that countered it for the psalmist.

Later I would understand how integrally bound up our reading and spirituality really are — how the thoughts that pass through our minds, urging them in this direction or that, become the very stuff of our inner beings, wedding us to God and everything around us. But for the time being there was a half-sensual, half-spiritual appeal in the words themselves, and I frolicked among them like a young Pan piping and dancing his way through a flowery meadow.

⌐⌐

Graduate school in English and American literature was a forest of endless delights. I was preaching to farmers in a country church every weekend and feasting the rest of the week on such writers as Browning, Tennyson, Wallace Stevens, Thomas Wolfe, and James Branch Cabell. I didn't ever quote what I was reading in my Sunday sermons. I don't know that I could do it even now with people who had read as little as my parishioners in that small church. But I was continually steeping myself in such delights as the poetry of John Donne and the fiction of John Steinbeck.

When I was reading Hemingway I noticed a strong parallelism between his personal philosophy, particularly about facing death, and that of the existentialists Heidegger, Jaspers, Sartre, and Camus, whom I was also

reading. Could I possibly write my Ph.D. dissertation on the way Hemingway's stories and novels closely mirrored the writings of the European
existentialists? My thesis committee agreed that it was a subject worth
pursuing, so I was off and running.

One of my professors, a dear, erudite man named Hill Shine, who taught
Victorian literature, took me aside one day and suggested that it would
be more appropriate for an aspiring young minister to write on one of
the English metaphysical poets or Sir Thomas Browne, the author of *Re-
ligio Medici*. He himself was an Episcopalian and an ardent student of
John Henry Newman, the nineteenth-century Anglican who converted
to Catholicism.

What I did was risky for a clergyman, I now realize. But it was also
crucial to my future penchant for finding new ways of relating the sacred
and the secular in a changing society. Hemingway attempted to write honestly — as honestly as he possibly could — and he was depicting a world
in which the chaos of World War I had changed everything, especially
among those who had fought in it. With the Europeans, in whose streets
and fields the war was waged, he experienced the absence of God in ways
we Americans would not know until the days of the Vietnam War and
the growth of a rebellious, secular culture.

This was very important for me to encounter, because I had never
been frontally exposed to real agnosticism before, or at least not in such
a way that I recognized it or had to grapple with it. And when I saw how
Hemingway and the European existentialists handled life without God —
their sense of living honorably, giving aesthetic shape to life, and refusing
to surrender to despair merely because the God of Western civilization
had died, as Nietzsche announced — I had my first real understanding of
what it means to millions of people today to live in the aftermath of a
dominant faith rather than in its heyday.

I no longer read Hemingway. I used to teach him — especially *The Old
Man and the Sea*, which is one of the most beautiful, mythopoeic books ever
written. But I think we have come far beyond him and his sense of what is

heroic in a de-divinized society. Now we have John Updike, who grapples with the heroism — or lack of it — in a man like Rabbit Angstrom, the frustrated ex-basketball player who became a car dealer, or Roger Lambert, the sad, unbelieving divinity-school professor of *Roger's Version*. Updike's people don't struggle with war and the virtues of manhood. They wrestle against invisible powers and principalities in a world where they are almost completely starved for meaning and relationship. They are Jake Barnes (Hemingway's famous protagonist in *The Sun Also Rises*) in the age of the Cold War and its aftermath, in the world of technology and impersonalism, when even the concept of manhood has evaporated and advertising jingles have triumphed over faith and philosophy.

٭

Over the years, I have been touched, moved, and rearranged by many poets and writers, and certain lines, scenes, and images come back at the oddest moments to provide captions for what is currently happening. Earlier today I was thinking about my own publishing and how honest I have tried to be in everything I have written. It reminded me of Samuel Beckett's spare little play *Waiting for Godot*, and how Beckett chose Roger Blin to direct it. Blin was preparing one of Strindberg's plays for production in Paris, and adhering strictly to the author's stage directions, despite the fact that it would probably make the play unpopular. Beckett went to see the play. Finding few people in the theater, he decided that Blin could be trusted to direct his own play.

I think about writers and their books that have had a seminal effect on me across the years. T. S. Eliot's *Murder in the Cathedral*. Dostoevsky's *The Brothers Karamazov*. Camus' *The Plague*. Kazantzakis' *Zorba the Greek* and *Report to Greco*. Annie Dillard's *Pilgrim at Tinker Creek*. Frederick Buechner's *The Final Beast* and *The Alphabet of Grace*. D. T. Suzuki's *Zen and Japanese Culture*. The novels, short stories, and letters of Flannery O'Connor. The poetry of Yeats, Hopkins, Auden, and Roethke. The plays of Ionesco, Albee, and Shaffer. Especially Shaffer.

It is interesting to note that I have not mentioned a single theological book. I have always read theology, of course — Barth, Tillich, Küng, Gilkey, Hick, Harvey Cox — and a number of biblical critics. But I realize that I have always found deeper meaning in novels and plays than in religious writings. There everything is still in its natural setting, without the designs and configurations imposed on it by some scholar's theories. I know it is a lot to say, but I would rather have written Brendan O'Carroll's *The Young Wan,* the affecting story of Agnes Brown, a girl who grows up in the Jarro, an inner-city area of Dublin, than John Calvin's *Institutes* or Karl Barth's *Church Dogmatics.* There is more durable truth in that one novel than in all the theological volumes I have ever read.

I have always liked and agreed with Buechner's assessment in *The Alphabet of Grace* that "at its heart, most theology, like most fiction, is essentially autobiography. Aquinas, Calvin, Barth, Tillich, working out their systems in their own ways and in their own language, are all telling us the stories of their lives, and if you press them far enough, even at their most cerebral and forbidding, you find an experience of flesh and blood, a human face smiling or frowning or weeping or covering its eyes before something that happened once. What happened once may be no more than a child falling sick, a thunderstorm, a dream, and yet it made for the face and inside the face a difference which no theology can ever entirely convey or entirely conceal."[1]

For me, the story behind the theology is far more interesting and exciting than the theology itself, for it is the flesh and blood, not the conclusions they prompted, that really compel our attention and arouse our compassion. The theology is only a construct, and, as such, is bound to lose its elasticity and harden into a pattern that one day no longer fits the facts of people's daily existence. But the stories behind the theologies — ah, those never lose their appeal, never cease to beg sympathy, never ossify into something subhuman or irrelevant, as the analytical works will do.

⌐

I am reading a great deal these days in the subject of world religions. I studied several major religions in divinity school at Harvard, and found them only vaguely interesting. But now I am fascinated by them, for I realize, as I didn't then, that there is far more similarity and continuity among all religions than I once noticed. The day is coming, I am convinced, when there will be a much greater amalgamation of the various faiths than we see today. I am not sure I would want them all to become alike, any more than I have ever wished the nations of Europe to become homogenized and speak the same language, because the world would lose so much color and quaintness if they did. But we shall one day acknowledge how the different belief systems fade and bleed into one another, forming a beautiful patchwork quilt of spiritual understanding.

I am also reading a lot of books my wife has told me about over the years, books I thought I didn't have time to read when I first heard her mention them. Books by women that I assumed were fine for entertainment but not really serious, the way some people once regarded George Eliot's *Mill on the Floss,* Jane Austen's *Pride and Prejudice,* Emily Brontë's *Wuthering Heights,* and Flannery O'Connor's *A Good Man Is Hard to Find.* I admit I was wrong. Now I am totally hooked on the novels of P. D. James, Maeve Binchy, Barbara Delinsky, Elizabeth Goudge, Rosamunde Pilcher, Anne Perry, and other fine women novelists of our time.

I fashioned the title of this book, in fact, after Rosamunde Pilcher's *Winter Solstice,* a story set in her native Scotland and told with such grace and elegance that I have wanted to return to Scotland ever since reading it and spend years steeping in that old culture. That's the thing about Pilcher's writing, I find. There are few great quotable passages in it, taken alone; but in the whole it is so provocative, so alluring, drawing the reader into a background as charming and exotic as if it were set in Kenya or Malaysia and not in the British Isles, that one adores it, luxuriates in it, and actually wants to reside in the houses where the characters live, eat the very meals they consume, and stroll on the beaches where they walk.

And that's the thing about stories, as opposed to books of theology and criticism — they open their doors and take us inside their vistas, so that we live what their characters live, see what they see, feel what they feel. And as Wordsworth said about poetry, thinking about them by some fantastic alchemy brings them alive in our minds, with the result that we actually experience the things they depict and those things become part of us. In that way they broaden our horizons and deepen our understanding. We become grander persons for every important book we read, for every sensitive poem over which we brood.

ᴄ⸴ᴐ

The variety of experiences in books, plays, and poetry, whether about world religions or domestic life in Scotland, enlarges our vision of life and teaches us to value it more than we did. If we go through life with our hands held open, so much more will fall into them than if we go with our hands closed and in our pockets. I am immeasurably enriched by everything I have read and heard and experienced through others, and I cannot imagine the life I take into my elder years without the benefit of all those glorious additions.

I can understand how this kind of openness alarms some of my old re-ligious friends, who think I have gone overboard in so many directions — Zen Buddhism, secular literature, immersion in foreign cultures — that I am hopelessly adrift from my moorings in the Christian faith. But I find that the greatest saints in Christian history, those with the truest and highest instincts, have always been most hospitable to people of other tra-ditions. Thomas Merton, for example, was in Thailand studying Buddhism when he died. Apparently he hoped to deepen his own already-profound prayer life by exposing it to that of his Asian friends.

For many years now, I have had a single test for the truth or reliability of a religious doctrine. If it promotes unity, and helps to bring people together in love and understanding, then it is true. If it does not, and ends by separating people, then it is false, regardless of how deeply embedded it is in tradition or how widely supported as a way of faith.

My bookshelves now reflect my predilection for acceptance and openness of spirit. Above my computer, arranged in no particular order on a single shelf, are such titles as *A History of God, The Coming of the Cosmic Christ, God and the Evolving Universe, The River of God, The Soul's Religion, The New American Spirituality, The Soul's Code, Teachings on Love, Visions of a New Earth, Belief in God in an Age of Science, A History of Time, Honest to Jesus,* and *Spiritual But Not Religious.* And behind me, clustered in a convenient area, are some of the writers I have for years found most refreshing and compatible with my own spirit: Annie Dillard, Loren Eiseley, Frederick Buechner, Nikos Kazantzakis, Carl Jung, Henri Nouwen, Gerard Manley Hopkins, Thomas Moore, Kathleen Norris, Matthew Fox, and D. T. Suzuki. If we are known by the company we keep, then I am happy to be known — even branded — by these writers.

☙

I realize, now that I am past seventy, that the "voice" in my writing has never been entirely my own. It has felt like mine, for I have always used it with confidence and been prepared to stand behind whatever it said. But merely talking about the writings that have been most significant to me across the years is enough to remind me that I have never spoken alone. Behind everything I have ever written or said there have been other voices, and behind theirs, still others, and behind theirs, yet again others, in an unbroken chain back through the ages. I suppose I am a Jungian about that — that there really is a collective unconscious, and that we know things from previous eras of history that we aren't always aware of knowing. Things that seep to the surface when we begin to think about matters or write about them. Things that came into our minds from God only knows where, linking us to various personalities in the past — ancient Greeks, Romans, Egyptians, Samoans, Scandinavians, whoever. It doesn't pay to be too fiercely independent — or too proud of our independence —

because our best thoughts and highest insights may actually be derived from someplace else. As my old friend and mentor Paul Scherer liked to say, "The ancients stole all our best ideas."

This telescoping of knowledge and understanding, Jung's notion that all living intelligence is connected to all other intelligence, whether human or animal, is the reason I have found Joanne Rowling's Harry Potter stories so fascinating. Rowling studied comparative literature and saw the telescoping at work in the writings of Homer, Virgil, Malory, Rabelais, Cervantes, Shakespeare, and all the great writers of the ages. And when she began crafting her brilliant stories about a young boy with powers of wizardry, she made him a lovable antihero with adumbrations of traits from all the great heroic literature of the past, including the Bible.

I had not read ten pages into the first volume, *Harry Potter and the Sorcerer's Stone*, when I exclaimed, "Why, Harry is a Christ figure!" It was so obvious. He was an orphan being brought to live in a world where he wasn't wanted. Supernatural manifestations occurred around him — there was an abundance of owls flying everywhere, and a downpour of shooting stars, and Dumbledore and McGonagall hovered over his arrival like the angels of God. Hagrid, the lumbering, red-faced gamekeeper who brought him, resembled nature and the elements. Harry had already been wounded, and bore a lightning-shaped scar on his forehead. There were nefarious forces actively seeking his destruction.

So when I began reading about Christians who rejected the Potter stories on the grounds that they would teach children to love witchcraft instead of God, I could not help writing *God, the Devil, and Harry Potter*. It was natural to me, instinctive, as most of my writing has been. It was something I had to say, that whether Rowling realized it or not (for such things can be unconscious to an author) she had assumed the entire Christian faith as a backdrop to her series, and was contributing to the Christ legend in literature as much as C. S. Lewis, J. R. R. Tolkien, and Charles Williams ever dreamed of doing.

Harry was an unwitting Christ-figure. Dumbledore was God the Father. His amazing phoenix, Fawkes (humorously named after Guy Fawkes, the insurrectionist whose effigy is burned in Britain on November 5 each year), was the Holy Spirit, always described as crimson and gold, like a fire. McGonagall, for Catholic readers, was a hovering mother-figure. Harry had a little band of inner disciples — Ron, Hermione, and Neville. In the very first novel, Harry descended into the underworld to slay the basilisk, a veritable symbol of evil, and then lay three days in a coma. Throughout the novels, he battled constantly against Lord Voldemort, the evil wizard whose bidding was done by ambitious clerks and nefarious bureaucrats.

Harry had his faults, as the religious fundamentalists have been quick to point out — he sometimes lied under pressure, was often disobedient, and invariably took shortcuts to reach desired ends. But he was always loving and considerate toward his friends, and faithful to a fault. In a world that could easily be described as apocalyptic, he lived as the dauntless champion of righteousness.

The Harry Potter series has charmed some people and deeply upset others. But we need to hear one another's viewpoints, and with as much civility as possible, the way the members of any family need to hear what all the others are thinking and feeling. Truth is never achieved unilaterally. It is something we all need to work at together and respectfully.

I regret the extraordinary one-sidedness with which Christianity tends to be reported and publicized in our country today. Sometimes I stand before the religion sections at Borders or Books-a-Million or Barnes and Noble and try to find the books that are openly expressive of unique or counter-viewpoints. Usually there are five or six authors and titles that fall into this category — among hundreds that represent the orthodox or conservative position. Only two or three major publishing houses today appear venturous enough to publish the works of more radical or out-spoken authors. All the others play it safe, politically and financially, by supporting the majority viewpoint. This makes me sad and furious. Truth is allowed the freedom to run — but only in shackles.

Yet I must not take all of this too seriously. From time to time, truth rises again and temporarily casts off its chains. Things are constantly mutating. This just happens to be a bad time for independent religious thought. So I'll read my Emerson and Wordsworth and Bishop Spong and Matthew Fox — and wait. As long as there's a Harry Potter in the world, our view of things will still be heard. Who knows? Even now, the next enormous, world-shattering revolution of ideas may be germinating in some child's mind!

ᴄ⌐

I would like to come back for a moment to the subject of women's writings, for I realize that I was almost dismissive of them, or appeared to be, when I spoke about not reading the books my wife was reading. Whatever I may have thought during my busier years of engagement, I am now convinced that women are on the whole much better writers than men. I say on the whole, for there are always exceptions — people such as John Updike and Thomas Moore and Brendan O'Carroll. But generally speaking, I find women to be more graceful, more intuitive, more expressive, and more comprehensive than men.

I began to see this during the 1970s, when more and more women were finding their way into my seminary classes and they were almost invariably superior to the men. They brought to the classroom a finer sensibility, a penchant for getting at the underside of matters and exposing them with deftness and a disarming sense of care. They nurtured material as they dealt with it — actually left it warmer, fuller, and more meaningful than they had found it. The men, by contrast, tended to expose things by tearing them apart and leaving the pieces carelessly strewn about, like the contents of a drawer in which they had been rummaging for something.

Now, as I relish the books of Elizabeth Goudge, Rosamunde Pilcher, and Dora Saint (aka Miss Read), I find myself feeling deficient because I am equipped solely with a man's point of view and wishing that I could see the world as tenderly and lovingly as they do. Yet I also find, as I admit this deficiency, that my way of seeing is subtly but definitely changing, that I am *beginning* to see and feel things as they do. In my own writing, I sense a greater and greater attraction to the forms of fiction, where it isn't necessary to pose as an authority in order to have something worthy to say. In fiction one can live in constant amazement at the beauty and fullness of the world even if there are wicked and unattractive elements within it.

I have always heard that we become more androgynous as we grow older — that women become more like men and men more like women. I hope that is true, for we men could certainly use some of the softness, resilience, and compassion of our mothers, sisters, and wives. It is in fact a spiritual thing to become more androgynous, and to recognize an expansion of one's own gender capacities into the roles and feelings of the other sex. As we grow older, and discover more and more traits of the other sex in ourselves, they are signs of our closeness to God. At least, that's what I'm telling myself these days.

〜

In the end, I find it quite impossible to imagine my life apart from everything I have read or absorbed from the culture without reading it. The great libraries of the world enrich our existence beyond all description, sensitizing us to infinite possibilities that we could never have dreamed for ourselves. They layer the world with plots, ideas, and characterizations, so that, if the world is indeed God's body, as Sallie McFague has insisted, it is a body so steeped in intellectual and emotional contrivances that we move about in it as if wading in some incredibly deep feather ticking, bouncing and floating and rejoicing like cherubs at play.

My sensibilities, apart from the authors I've read, would be extremely limited, like those of an aborigine or perhaps some unusually intelligent animal. But as it is they are expanded and honed by hosts of remarkable persons, from Geoffrey Chaucer to Saul Bellow and Emily Dickinson to Elie Wiesel, so that I have been able to live vicariously in many times and places I didn't actually inhabit, and see life through the eyes of characters as widely divergent as Falstaff and Lear, Dorian Gray and Jude Fawley, Jane Eyre and Zorba the Greek. And I can't help feeling that, because I have this wider range of sympathy and understanding, I know more about the mind of God and am able to pray with a greater assurance of somehow being a mystical part of that mind.

Books, in other words, have been a large part of my continuing conversion.

Five

The Joy of
Honest Work

As I hinted earlier, work has always been for me a form of play, something I become so caught up in and enjoy so much that it doesn't seem to be work at all. All work should really be that way. I still like the title of Marsha Sinetar's book *Do What You Love, the Money Will Follow*. I'm not sure the money does follow, at least not when it's most needed. It didn't for Van Gogh, and it hasn't for a lot of people I know, especially artists and musicians and writers. It didn't always for me.

But the idea of doing what one loves — as one's work or calling — is very important to me. I have always believed that the surest way to waste a life would be to spend it working at things one didn't like, even if the things looked very appropriate to the world, such as practicing medicine, chairing a Fortune 500 company, or emerging as a major political figure. When our children were growing up we always insisted that it was all right for them to become anything they liked — even street cleaners, park attendants, or dish washers — as long as they were happy and found fulfillment in what they were doing.

Later, when we watched other people's children becoming doctors, lawyers, and bankers, and our sons were still floundering about in art and academics and not really earning a living, we wondered if we had overdone it. But I still maintain that a life spent working at something that gives one a sense of having made the world more loving, more beautiful, or more peaceful is to be preferred to any life that is lived merely to create wealth, command attention, or satisfy a desire for power and celebrity.

c—ɔ

I think I have always loved to work, even when I was a child.

When I was ten, I accompanied my father on his business trips into the country and bought watermelons from farmers at ten cents each. Then I peddled them from door to door in my little wooden wagon and sold them for fifty and seventy-five cents apiece, depending on their size.

At eleven, I became a caddy at the local golf course, and was thrilled, on a Saturday afternoon when I could carry two bags instead of one, to earn as much as three or four dollars.

When I was twelve I took a paper route with the *Courier Journal,* our state's most prestigious newspaper. It wasn't merely one paper route, it was two, as the boy who had had it eventually acquired an extra route. We lived on the highway north of town, and the paper truck bearing the papers from Louisville came roaring past our house about four o'clock every morning. I always set my alarm, got up, dressed, and waited until I heard the truck go by. Then I walked a mile up the dark road to the little service station where my papers were dropped off last, after the others had been left at the central office.

Being a paperboy was a wonderful experience in business, for it quickly taught me that while some people are honest, there are others who are simply deadbeats and will try to avoid paying what they owe, even for newspapers. I operated on a slender margin of profit. Of the thirty-five cents people paid for a week's worth of papers, I kept only eleven cents. If three customers failed to pay in a given week, it cut into my profits by 10 percent. So I quickly learned to be resourceful. If customers didn't pay on Saturday morning, when I covered the route a second time to collect, I hammered on their doors when I brought the paper on Sunday. This was usually between six and seven o'clock, before most people had risen, so it was a very effective way of getting them to pay. If customers went for more than two weeks without paying, I stopped delivery. Then I would get irate calls demanding to know where their papers were and I would explain my policy. After the first month, I had little trouble collecting.

In some ways it was a lonely experience walking a paper route before dawn. But it was also a beautiful time, when everything was ghostly quiet, the air was clean and fresh, and, as I was finishing up and heading home, the first bright rays of the sun were just beginning to illuminate the world. Sometimes I talked to myself as I walked, and sometimes I talked to God. I took great pride in folding the papers neatly and placing them exactly where people wanted to find them. Although I was only twelve, I felt that I was already becoming a responsible servant in my community.

Few people tipped the paperboy in those days. Those who did usually gave me a nickel. Then there was Mrs. Ben Adkins, whose husband owned a candy distributorship. She was a nice lady with very prominent features, a beauty-parlor hairdo, and a slow Southern drawl, and she was active in local club life. Mrs. Adkins always complimented me on the fine job I was doing, and when she paid me she also gave me a candy bar as "a little something extra." Usually it was a Baby Ruth or a Powerhouse, neither of which I liked very much. And I don't remember ever getting one that wasn't already turning white with age.

I am confident that I never let on to that dear lady that I didn't really like the candy she gave me or that I knew she had either had it for a while or her husband had brought home outdated candy from the store. It was the beginning of a lifetime of being kind and polite to people even when I knew they were trying to put one over on me, which came in very handy as training for the Christian ministry.

In the summer of my thirteenth year I had more energy than my two paper routes could satisfy, so I undertook another task. My mother had become an insurance agent, and every afternoon she had to go to the courthouse to look up the motor numbers of the vehicles she had insured that day. As I sometimes accompanied her, I noticed that the other agents had to do the same thing. What if they had a list of all the motorists in the county, I wondered, complete with their addresses, vehicle information, and motor numbers? Confident that the agents would be happy to buy such a list, I spent most of that summer in the clerk's office copying information onto yellow legal pads, then producing multiple copies on an old Underwood typewriter when I got home. Those were the days before copy machines as we know them, so I typed several "first" copies and made four or five carbons with each. Of course this meant a laborious process whenever I made a mistake, rolling the pages forward, separating them, rubbing the erroneous letter or numeral with a special typewriter eraser, blowing away the gritty rubbings, and then carefully restoring the pages to their original position. But by summer's end I had produced about thirty copies of the precious document, which I easily sold for twenty-five dollars apiece. It was more money than I expected to make in a lifetime!

The next year my father and mother opened an Army-Navy surplus store, and I had a regular job after school and on Saturdays clerking in the store. I have always believed that whatever people skills I possess derived principally from that early experience of dealing with all kinds of customers in a retail store. I learned to value the poor people who dug deeply into their pockets to purchase surplus socks or shoes as much as I did the many wealthier farmers, contractors, and professional people who purchased large equipment such as winches, generators, and cranes.

I also learned to have real confidence in myself, especially after customers began asking for me to wait on them. I had a quick mind for the location of every item in the store — more often than not I had placed it there myself — and for the prices of literally everything. I became adept at pointing out the qualities of the items I was selling and, if there was any confusion in the customer's mind, recommending one item over another. I was invariably cheerful and helpful, and gladly went the second mile to assist people with their purchases. Many customers were amazed that I was as strong as I was, lifting great coils of rope or cable and helping to load such heavy items as gasoline engines or large tarpaulins. But I felt as if I had the strength of ten, because I enjoyed what I was doing.

Confirming my entrepreneurial bent, I developed an extra business in addition to working at my parents' store. For several months I had been selling minnows to local fishermen. I seined the little creek below our house to get the minnows, often coming home with thirty or forty large chubs at a time. But it soon became apparent that there was a call for more minnows than I could supply, as the gradual formation of a new lake in the area was attracting many out-of-town fishermen. I then contracted with a minnow farm near Junction City, Kentucky, to supply as many minnows as I could sell.

I kept the minnows in an old spring box where the water was always cool and fresh. It had a corrugated tin roof, with a cable running through a pulley and a dead weight on the other end, so that I could raise or lower it to any height and it would stay there until I moved it again.

For most of that summer I sold several hundred minnows a week. As many of my customers wanted to get to the lake before dawn, I made appointments to dip up their minnows at three or four in the morning, and therefore didn't lose any time working at the store. And as I paid only a penny for each minnow and sold it for five cents, I was making what seemed to me a great deal of money.

Late in the summer, however, disaster struck. A bacterial infection began forming mucous on the minnows' lungs and gills. Each morning I would find dozens of dead minnows floating on the water. I stopped selling minnows for a week, during which I drained the spring box and scrubbed it out with a detergent. But the blight was persistent, and eventually I gave up the business. I couldn't stand the deaths of all those little creatures!

༕

I have sometimes wondered where I got my sense of industry. Was it from the genes of ancestors similarly dedicated to work? Was it from boredom in our little community, where the movies changed once a week and church was the only other venue of entertainment? Was it from a desire to make money? Or was it from the need to prove myself, especially to a father whose approval I never seemed to have?

Perhaps it was the last reason, if any of these was correct. But the truth is that I always enjoyed working and felt recharged by it. The achievements didn't have to be prodigious. I derived pleasure from doing little things — mowing the grass, trimming the shrubs, building a bookcase, writing letters, washing and polishing the car — as much as big ones.

But maybe there's another reason I grew up liking to work. It was during those years that I was having my adolescent experiences of spirituality. The God I knew about then was a creator — he had made the world and everything in it. My religion glorified work. With a history in the Reformed tradition going back to the Puritans themselves, it commended busyness over idleness and industry over lethargy: "Idle hands are the devil's workshop." I heard that *bon mot* many times. So perhaps I was doing something religious when I worked. I'm not sure. I played with equal zeal, and my religion didn't recommend that. But I probably did feel a sense of righteousness about my working. It was something to be proud of.

What is it like to work? Abraham Maslow's idea of the "peak experience," the moment when our activities coincide so beautifully with our energies and abilities that we virtually *hum* at what we are doing, is as apt a way of describing it as I know. I remember a poem by Jane Mayhall in *The New Yorker* entitled "Painkiller." She said that work is an anesthetic that connects with our neurological tracks to produce an "aprodisiacal forgetfulness." Maybe so, but work was always more than that for me. As far back as I can remember, working was a transcendent activity, one in which I managed to "slip the surly bonds of earth," as the hymn puts it, and soar into a stratosphere of excitement and pleasure. In a sense, I suppose, it is a game one plays against oneself, always trying to win by doing better and achieving more than one expected. When I really hit my stride in whatever I am doing — pushing a lawnmower, shoveling mulch, carrying firewood, painting window trim, writing a book — I am as absorbed and captivated as if I were playing tennis or hiking a mountain trail. I'm releasing endorphins like crazy, and I'm intoxicated with the project at hand. I am on a high, and don't fully come down for some time after I finish.

Is there anything spiritual about this? Of course there is. It all has to do with energy. The Spirit of God is pure energy. When energy flows through us, we are experiencing a transcendent presence. The problem with many people's lives — the reason they are frustrated and unhappy — is that they have not learned to channel energy. The energy they have, or might have, is bottled up inside them and can't discharge itself through their activities. Hence they become conflicted and joyless.

☙

My capacity to work served me well through my years of education and in my career as a minister and teacher. Looking back now, I can see the pattern. I *was* my work. My work was always an expression of the inner me, just as surely as if I had been a finalist at Wimbledon, an Oscar-winning actor, or a well-known public figure. I produced it as naturally, and in some ways almost as effortlessly, as a spider emits its web, weaving an effect of wonder and mystery.

Nobody ever told me I should work hard in school. I simply found that learning and growing were fun. In high school English classes, I enjoyed writing extra themes, often with humorous or mock-serious undertones. I studied the dictionary to develop an effective vocabulary, because I discovered that knowing words allowed me to have ideas I wouldn't otherwise have had. My professors in graduate school liked having me in their classes because I mirrored back their own excitement and comprehension when they talked about their favorite subjects. Sometimes they embarrassed me by reading my papers or examination essays to the rest of the class and commending them as models. Years later, when I returned to the University of Kentucky for a Phi Beta Kappa award, the presenter identified herself as someone who had been in one of my classes and had been awed by what I appeared to know and how much reverence my professors accorded me.

Reflecting on her remarks, I had to admit that I was completely unaware of such a status in the eyes of my fellow students or of any special deference from the teachers. I was simply in love with what I was doing and felt that immersing myself in it was the only thing to do. I was enthralled, and when I am enthralled I never know how hard I am working. It is still the same today.

Speaking of "immersing" reminds me of my parallel life in the church while I was acquiring my college and graduate-school education. I worked very hard at that too, and was as fully absorbed in doing my best there as I was in the classroom. In my first parish, when I was eighteen, I soon recruited a group of twenty people who wanted to be baptized and join the congregation. In the Baptist church, baptism was, of course, by a single mode — immersion. As our building didn't have a baptismal pool, we had to borrow one at another Baptist church on a Sunday evening. It was my first experience of baptizing anyone, although I had witnessed the ritual many times. The pastor of the church was very kind, and loaned me his baptismal boots and robe for the occasion. The boots were like fishing waders, reaching all the way to the chest. When I put them on, I took off my suit coat and shoes, but left my shirt and wool trousers on.

The baptisms went very well — I was really getting the hang of it — until the very end. After immersing all the candidates, I raised my arms from the baptismal pool to give the benediction. The minister had failed to remind me to fasten the rubber cuffs in the sleeves of the robe to make them watertight. When I raised my arms, several quarts of water were scooped up in the sleeves and cascaded down into the rubber boots, completely soaking my shirt and trousers.

I rode back to college in wet clothes, and shivered as I walked a mile through the wintry night from the bus stop to the house where I lived. The next day I came down with a terrible cold!

~⁊

My energy level then, as now, was extremely high. My wife accuses me of always wanting to do things on a skateboard, where it is necessary to stay fully absorbed in order to remain vertical. I graduated from college at the age of nineteen. Four years later, I had earned my first doctorate. While I was writing my doctoral thesis at the University of Kentucky I took courses in Greek and theology at Lexington Theological Seminary, so that I was able to complete my three-year degree program at Harvard Divinity School in only two years.

During the summer between my graduation from the university and my matriculation at Harvard, I needed to make some money before leaving for Massachusetts. The employment agency offered two possibilities. One was to be an extra in a movie called *State Fair,* starring Pat Boone, that was to be filmed on location in the Bluegrass. The other was to be a salesman at a Baker's Qualicraft Shoe Store. The work at the shoe store was hard because the shoes sold for only three or four dollars a pair and salaries were based solely on commission. This meant waiting on two or three customers simultaneously in order to make any money at all. But I figured the movie would be good for only four to six weeks of work, while I could keep the job at the shoe store for the entire summer. If I really hustled, I could make a lot more money selling shoes. So that's what I did.

(Many years later, I became president of an organization called the Mission for Biblical Literacy and asked Pat Boone to serve on the board of directors. Happily, he accepted the position with enthusiasm. I don't think I ever mentioned to him that I almost appeared in one of his movies!)

After working my way through college and graduate school — always with Anne's help — I had hoped to spend my first year at Harvard concentrating on my studies and not having to work. But it soon became apparent that the Boston area was too expensive for that. So, two months after we arrived, I became minister of the Martin's Pond Union Baptist Church in North Reading, Massachusetts, a few miles north of Boston. The salary was two thousand dollars a year and we were given a furnished parsonage with all our utilities paid. We thought we were in tall clover!

While I was at Harvard, Anne spent her time studying piano under Jeannette Giguere at the New England Conservatory of Music. Each week she earned two dollars by cleaning the church and used that money to purchase any music she wasn't able to copy by hand. We both worked hard in New England, but had a wonderful time in that exotic setting and have always considered it one of the finest periods of our lives.

Have I ever wished I hadn't driven myself so relentlessly during those years and had taken more time to enjoy things? Of course. But I wouldn't take anything for what I learned or the people I met and worked with. Given the choice, I'd probably do the same thing all over again. They were glorious, exciting years, and I look back on them now with a lot of gratitude. Besides, at the time, I had the wonderful feeling that I was doing everything for God. Working to get where I was going was my service to him.

The professional years that followed were also filled with lots of wonderful, absorbing work, and again with the sense that I was doing it for God.

When I left Harvard, I wanted to return to the South. But I found that most Baptist churches were unprepared to receive a minister who had studied at Harvard; they felt safer with ministers trained in their own seminaries. So I took a position as a professor of English at Georgetown College in Kentucky, which I had attended for a year as an undergraduate. I figured that God would eventually straighten things out and get me into a pastorate, but in the meantime I would do my best at the employment I could get.

I still laugh about the dilemma I faced at that time. Ph.D.'s in English were scarce at private institutions, where salaries were lower than at state universities. Therefore I was offered a position at Union University in Tennessee as chairman of the English department, even though I had never taught a day in my life, at a salary of forty-five hundred dollars a year. Georgetown offered an associate professorship with a salary of five thousand dollars. I was happy to forego the honor of a chairmanship for the extra five hundred dollars!

I don't think I ever lived as close to the edge of happy exhaustion as I did during my two years at Georgetown. The first year, I had five classes each semester, including two freshman English classes that required marking countless student themes. Keeping ahead of my classes in textbooks that were new to me, preparing for my lectures, and marking all those papers made me burn the midnight oil almost every night. And on the weekends I was usually off to preach somewhere.

My second year at Georgetown I was made dean of the chapel — God was moving me toward the pastorate! — and charged with upgrading the college's religious services. My course load was accordingly reduced to nine hours, but I still labored devotedly, knowing how much the success of the program hinged on my having good prayers and sermons every week. Dr. George Redding, the distinguished head of the Bible department, once told a colleague during one of those services, who repeated it to me, that the students didn't know it, but they were hearing some of the best preaching in America. I have always been grateful for that remark.

Not all of my life at Georgetown was work, of course. It was during this second year that our first son, John Eric, was born, and I didn't miss a day of the magic of that beautiful event. The whole affair — Anne's pregnancy, her growing belly, the baby's kicks, the birth, the nighttime changing and feedings (which I handled because Anne was temporarily indisposed), and all the joys of a first child after nine years of marriage without one — was fully as engrossing as my life in the college.

⌇

Shortly afterward we went off to Princeton, where I had been invited to come for a year as assistant to the distinguished preacher Dr. Paul E. Scherer. Former minister of Holy Trinity Lutheran Church in New York and professor of homiletics at Union Theological Seminary, Scherer taught at Princeton several years after retiring from New York. We went expecting to stay only a year. But Dr. Scherer pleaded with me to stay another year — he didn't want to lose his grader — and said I could use a book I was writing, *The Failure of Theology in Modern Literature*, as my thesis for a doctor-of-theology degree.

Given such an enticement, I could hardly afford to leave. I was an instructor in preaching at the seminary, had a lucrative Rockefeller Fund scholarship, and was minister of the young Raritan Valley Baptist Church in nearby Edison, New Jersey. My combined income was more than twice what I had been making at Georgetown. So I stayed another year and took a doctorate in homiletics and liturgics. That meant sitting for the exams, which of course required a great deal of reading and preparation, but it seemed a small price to pay for a Princeton doctorate.

When the time came to return to Georgetown, which had extended my leave of absence for the second year, I was lured instead to a new college in Louisville called Kentucky Southern College. It too was a Baptist school, but one founded with very advanced educational ideas and aspirations. I was attracted by the visionary president, Dr. Rollin Burhans, and the college's commitment to interdisciplinary studies. Because I now had doctorates in both English and theology, Dr. Burhans wanted me to be the academic dean of the institution — I was supposed to be a living example of interdisciplinary studies — and promised me free rein in both curricular design and the hiring of faculty. That was heady stuff, and I was too young and inexperienced to know how inadequately prepared I was to manage it. I think I did a good job — I certainly gave it my all — even though most of what I accomplished more or less vanished when Kentucky Southern later merged with the University of Louisville.

Among the things I learned during my brief tenure as a dean was that I did not like administrative work, mainly because it required an endless round of meetings. I was already beginning to receive invitations to become president of this or that college, but knew that a president's schedule is as impacted as a dean's. Besides, I still felt a commitment to preaching and the church. So when I had an opportunity to go to Vanderbilt University to teach preaching in the divinity school, I was happy to take a huge salary cut and go. I felt that I was getting my life back, and my family's as well. I also believed God was moving me closer to the pastorate.

Teaching in a divinity school was probably the easiest, least-demanding thing I ever did. To begin with, the school year was actually only eight months long, with generous holidays at Christmas and Easter. My teaching load was light — two courses one semester and three the next. I could choose the courses myself. Nobody ever asked to see a course plan, so I was free to design them any way I wished. And, on top of everything else, we were encouraged to take frequent sabbatical leaves.

The one pressure at Vanderbilt was to publish. But that was a snap. I had recently published not one book but three, and thought I had the hang of it. And with all the free time I had, writing books was a cinch. In one year, 1973, I had five books come out from different publishers. *The Nashville Tennessean* ran a cover story on me in its Sunday rotogravure section, describing me as a publishing machine.

In addition to teaching and writing, I soon became a frequent flier on the lecture circuit, zipping all over the U.S. and sometimes even abroad to speak at church conferences, university gatherings, and military retreats. I hated being gone so much, because I missed Anne and our two sons. (Our second son, Paul Krister, was born while we lived in Louisville.) But the revenue from this extra work paid our sons' tuition in an excellent private school and allowed us to make frequent summer trips abroad.

While I did not regard all the busyness during those years as especially taxing, I can look back now and see that I sometimes pushed the envelope. Once, when I was lecturing at Wake Forest University in North Carolina,

I had a terrible pain in my side that turned out to be a severe muscle spasm. When I got home, our doctor friend, Edward Benz, gave me some muscle relaxants and advised me to take it easy for a while. Ed knew that I had a hard time hearing such advice. Even when I went on sabbatical leave for a year, I always produced at least two or three books.

c-ɔ

In 1976, the Plymouth Congregational Church in Minneapolis, Minnesota, one of the most progressive congregations in America, approached me about becoming their senior minister. My family and I drove to Minneapolis to see the church and meet with their search committee. I was strongly tempted — perhaps God was finally going to give me a church to pastor. In addition to offering a salary considerably above the one I earned by teaching, the church had its own theater and its own circulating art gallery. It also sent its minister and his family on an annual trip around the world to check on its various academic and medical missions. Dr. Howard Conn, the erudite senior minister who was retiring, often packed the two-thousand-seat sanctuary with lectures on Plato and other well-known philosophers.

But after much soul-searching, I turned down the invitation. I had prayed and prayed about it, and didn't feel God calling me there. Six months later, the committee came back with added inducements. This time I weakened and said I would come. I hadn't been able to get the church off my mind. "But don't make the announcement yet," I cautioned. "Give me a couple of weeks to make sure I've made the right decision." At the end of two weeks, with calls almost every day from the search committee, I said, "No, I can't do it. I don't know why, but it doesn't feel right." God still hadn't said yes.

In the summer of 1977 my family and I went to Ireland for two weeks and then on to Oxford, where I would spend the year on sabbatical. I wrote three books that year: *The Loneliness of Children; Prayer: The Act of*

Being with God; and a novel called *Gentle, My Love* that a New York agent liked but was never able to place with a publisher.

For me personally, however, it was a year of inner turmoil. The invitation to Plymouth Church had stirred up something inside me that I couldn't stop thinking about. It was a midlife desire to return to the pastorate on a full-time basis. I thought God wanted me to be a preacher. Yet I was still teaching in a divinity school and hadn't felt right about going to Minneapolis. I wondered if I was going to have a breakdown.

I remember reading Sir Francis Chichester's *The Lonely Sea and the Sky* that year. Among Chichester's many exploits as an adventurer, the one that captivated me most was his extraordinary flight from New Zealand to Australia, a trip as perilous as Lindbergh's solo flight across the Atlantic. Chichester had his little plane *The Gipsy Moth* outfitted with extra petrol tanks, but, even so, needed to set down en route for refueling. He studied the map and chose tiny Falkland Island as his destination for this task.

Chichester had barely begun his journey when clouds filled the sky and high winds began sweeping him off course. The only thing he could do was wait until he spotted some sundogs where there was a break in the clouds, abandon his present course, fly into the break, take new bearings, and recalculate his direction.

This occurred again and again, greatly increasing the possibility that he would not be able to find Falkland Island and would perish in the sea.

When he finally reached the place where he figured the island should be, Chichester could see nothing but clouds. But he dipped his plane down under the clouds and there was the island, a beautiful emerald-green spot in the middle of the gray water. Feeling enormously relieved, he landed, refueled, and took off again for Australia.

That image, of Chichester being blown off course and having to take new bearings, spoke to me with tremendous force. I had set out with the objective of being a minister, and had been blown off course. Now I needed to find my way back. I decided that God did indeed want me to return to the parish ministry, and that the church in Minneapolis had been used to reignite my interest. We came back to the U.S. at the end of the year and I began searching for the church where I felt that God really wanted me to be.

My search led to conversations with several promising churches from Michigan to Texas and Virginia to California. I was greatly attracted to the glorious old First Congregational Church of Los Angeles, but learned that the congregation had had a history of fractiousness and worried that I didn't have enough experience in larger churches to handle the situation there. The First Presbyterian Church of Lynchburg, Virginia, on the other hand, appeared to be in excellent shape. It was a vigorous upper-middle-class church in the most beautiful part of a stately old city. The members got along well and had no history of internal clashes. So in the end I accepted the call to Virginia.

The Congregationalists in L.A. said, "OK, we understand. But we will hire an older minister who will be here for only a few years. When he retires, we'll call you again."

Probably no one but my wife and my secretary knew how hard I worked in Lynchburg the six years I was a minister there, or how happy I was doing it. In addition to the usual pastoral responsibilities of leading worship and preaching, recruiting new members, visiting the sick and elderly, burying the dead, consoling the living, and chairing the session (the major board of the church), I redesigned the worship service, taught classes in spirituality, initiated a Christmas Eve service for the bereaved, held leadership classes in sensitivity training, organized a lay visitation program for the sick and elderly, oversaw the writing and publication of a weekly newsletter, started an annual preaching mission that brought distinguished speakers to the church, began a program of work-release for prisoners, and imported some new staff members who had a galvanizing effect on the church's life and work.

The prayers, sermons, and other things I wrote inevitably found their way into several books. I also published two books about ministry, *The Tender Shepherd* and *Christ and the Seasons of Ministry*, and a preaching textbook called *Fundamentals of Preaching*. All of this during a six-year pastorate in which I was an active, hands-on minister who continued to lecture and preach in other parts of the country as well. I think about it now and wonder how in the world I managed to do it!

～

The people in California were as good as their word. On the day their senior minister retired, six years after we went to Lynchburg, they phoned to ask if I was ready to come to Los Angeles. I said yes; I could hardly wait. Six months later we were living in Hollywood.

If I had worked hard in Virginia, I found that it was necessary to work even harder in L.A. Just staying alive there wasn't easy. The streets were tough, the traffic was unbelievable, everything happened at lightning speed, the church faced even bigger problems than I had realized, and there were some perennially hostile members in the congregation who invariably opposed whatever came down the road, even if it looked like Jesus on a donkey. Before I had been there a whole month, I came home one night from a church council meeting and told Anne, "I've got to get out of here, honey, or it will kill me. But let's try to stay at least until the first of the year. That way it won't look so bad on my résumé."

Sometimes, as a kind of therapy, I made lists of all the things I had to do in the course of a single day. Here is a typical list, chosen at random and slightly modified to omit personal references:

Met with three trustees at breakfast

Went over week's schedule with secretary

Responded to letters and memos

Had planning session with associate ministers

Interviewed candidates for staff position

Wrote pastor's paragraph for weekly bulletin

Prepared Sunday prayers

Had lunch with Women's Association

Visited members in two different hospitals

Reviewed agenda for deacon's meeting

Returned phone calls

Met with a disgruntled member

Attended board meeting for HopeNet, Inc. (a hunger organization)

Took two phone calls during dinner

Met with board of deacons

It was hardly a cushy job, but my lists probably didn't look very different from the average CEO's. And one part of me actually thrived on such busyness. While much of it was management on the run, it really felt good to meet so many tasks head on and bring a semblance of order out of their potential chaos. That is probably what energizes most CEOs.

It wasn't the work that exhausted me at First Congregational Church of Los Angeles. It was the unusual amount of contentiousness among the members. A minister who had once had a long pastorate at the church, Dr. James W. Fifield Jr., had been a virtual potentate, and when he retired he left an enormous power vacuum. A number of strong-willed people, particularly several attorneys, had been contending for leadership roles ever since. They actually seemed to thrive on the conflicts they engendered. But they nearly drove me crazy! The worst part was that I never could feel that the church as a whole cared about serving God. It was only a grand old institution with no commitment to anything beyond itself.

We stayed three years at the First Congregational Church of Los Angeles — three exciting, demanding years that drained me more than any comparable period of my life. The church grew, the program improved, and so did the church's financial condition. And hopefully I was able to show at least some people the way to a deeper, more satisfying spiritual life. But after three years I was running on fumes. I simply couldn't bear the contentious atmosphere any longer. When Dr. Thomas Corts, the president of Samford University in Birmingham, Alabama, invited me to join Samford's faculty as Distinguished Professor of Religion and Culture, I saw it as a ladder let down out of heaven!

Unfortunately, as I learned later, that ladder didn't come from heaven. But I'll get to that in another chapter. For now I'll simply say that Samford offered a welcome change at the time, and I felt relieved at the chance to return to a university campus.

༄

I liked being back in the genteel hum of university life. As a distinguished professor, I was allowed to teach whatever I wished, and so offered courses in the new divinity school, the religion department, and the English department. I particularly relished the opportunity to teach a seminar in creative writing, and had a number of talented students who made our sessions very enjoyable. I was especially grateful for having more time to write and study, and began reviewing what I had learned in my parish experiences as the basis for a book called *Preaching to a Church in Crisis: A Homiletic for the Last Days of the Mainline Church.*

During my third year at Samford, I was asked to chair a committee charged with designing a special program for the university's sesquicentennial celebration. We called the program "Christfest" and made it a week-long celebration of Christianity and the arts. Several outstanding personalities were invited to take part in the festivities, including my former classmate from the University of Kentucky, the famous poet and ecologist Wendell Berry. The sleeper in the group was Father Joseph Girzone, a Catholic priest whose novels about Joshua, a contemporary Christ-figure, had been banned at the Vatican but had at the same time become the rage among evangelicals in this country.

Not knowing how Father Girzone would be accepted on a Baptist campus — it was the first time a Roman Catholic had ever spoken there — Anne and I invited him to stay at our home. Our time together led to a strong and lasting friendship. Before Joe left, I proposed that he come, live in our home for a few months, and write a Joshua novel set in the South, which, I tried to persuade him, has always been a matrix of religious passion. Joe's simple reply was, "I don't like grits." Then he explained that he was from New York and didn't think he could ever understand the South enough to construct a story about it.

"Why don't you write it?" he asked.

Those five words would prove to be very influential. A year later, I began working on *Jessie,* a novel about a female Christ-figure who is an artist and settles in the vicinity of Gatlinburg, Tennessee. And three or four years after that I would write a sequel, *The Night Jessie Sang at the Opry,* in which Jessie was a singer/song-writer living in Nashville.

⌒⌒

When Dr. Donald Ward, my predecessor at the First Congregational Church of Los Angeles, retired from that church, he became the minister of the Little Stone Church on Mackinac Island, Michigan, a seasonal church that was open from mid-May to early October. He told me that it was the jewel in the crown of all his experience as a minister, and he enjoyed it more than anything he had ever done.

But in April of 1994, Don called to say he had just learned that he had terminal cancer and would not be able to keep his summer contract with the congregation on the island. Could I possibly take his place, now that I was teaching in a university and had my summers off? I wanted to help Don and was tempted to do it, but unfortunately I already had a number of speaking commitments that would have interfered. Our son Eric, on the other hand, who was also an ordained minister, had recently become divorced and given up his parish, and I thought he would be available. A committee from the Little Stone Church accordingly interviewed him and called him to be their minister. He spent two happy summers at the church before remarrying and assuming another parish in Atlanta.

When Eric told the members at the Little Stone Church that he was leaving, they asked if I could come as their pastor. This time I was happy to say yes. Anne and I spent the next eight summers at the Little Stone Church, she as the organist and I as the minister. It was a very fulfilling experience for both of us, particularly because it was the only time since our early rural churches when we had been able to work as a team to lead worship services.

Inasmuch as the season on Mackinac extended into the month of October, while the university's academic year commenced in late August, I decided that it would be best to resign from my appointment at Samford. So, after a single year on the island, I tendered my resignation from the university and became officially semiretired. I would spend four and a half months a year preaching, performing weddings, and ministering to the people at Mackinac, and the other seven and a half writing, traveling, and enjoying life.

For the next several years that is what I did. Out of those years came some of the most important books — I believe — that I have written, including *God, the Devil, and Harry Potter; Raising Your Spiritual Awareness Through 365 Simple Gifts from God; Ten Things I Learned Wrong from a Conservative Church; Lost in Wonder, Love, and Praise;* and *Enter Every Trembling Heart.* My experiences as a pastor on an island also provided the background for a novel set on a fictional island, *Maggie Bowles and the Mystery of the Marigold Turtle.*

Looking back over what I have written in this chapter I am embarrassed at the preoccupation with myself and what I have done. Such preoccupation is natural, I suppose. We all tend to look back on the highlights of our careers and engage in at least minimal self-glorification. It's simply the way things work. For most of our careers, we try to sell ourselves, to make ourselves look important, employable, indispensable, and promotable. It is part of the onward-and-upward posture of the American workplace. And sometimes, as a result, we forget to make real distinctions between our CVs and our actual biographies — who we really are under the veneer.

The world teaches us to lead from our strengths and achievements. But God probably wants us to lead with our weaknesses and vulnerabilities. I feel guilty when I think of this. My mental checkups have usually been very self-congratulatory, as if I have done well for a person of my background and abilities. But if I had been more sensitive to my own spiritual understanding I might have had a lot more humility.

Occasionally, when asked for a PR sheet on myself, I have produced one that I consider at least partially honest. Here are some paragraphs from it: "Killinger has displayed a great deal of instability in his denominational orientation, having begun his career as a Baptist, attended a Disciples of Christ church, then become a Presbyterian and finally a Congregationalist. Those who know him best speculate that he may have a serious identity problem. Others say he merely wore out his welcome with each successive group and had to keep moving on.

"He has written a number of books, none of them memorable, and has been on the editorial boards of two undistinguished professional magazines, both of which flirted constantly with bankruptcy and eventually succumbed to it.

"The one honor in his lifetime that he thought was truly solid was when he was made an honorary citizen of Lubbock, Texas, by the mayor of that city, who was a member of a church where Killinger was speaking. But when Killinger returned to Lubbock several years later, nobody recognized him and the mayor's office was locked up and bore a "Gone Fishing" sign on the door.

"Killinger married above himself, to a lovely woman named Anne Kathryn who plays the piano and the organ and has written a few books herself, all better than his. Together they raised two sons, Eric and Krister, who are both smarter than their father and have a lot more sense about how to live and enjoy the world."

This may sound like a spoof. But in the end what are our achievements anyway, especially when compared with those of a Helen Keller, a Stephen Hawking, or a Martin Luther King Jr.? Most of us are like the fellow who was introduced as "a legend in his own mind." Our successes are mostly monuments to our own self-absorption, and of little real value to the world as a whole.

What is important about work is finally the joy and satisfaction it brings to our existence — the fact that we are able to do anything at all, and to do it with enough grace and panache to feel pleased about it. As for its place in God's kingdom — well, maybe it is like those barely recognizable portraits our children present to us when they're just learning to draw with crayons. God is pleased, not because we show talent, but because he loves us and enjoys seeing us get excited about what we can do.

⌒⌒

Several years ago, my longtime friend Dr. Wayne Oates, one of the originators of the pastoral care movement in America, wrote a book called *Confessions of a Workaholic*. For most of his life, he said, he had not realized that he was obsessed with work. Then, one summer when he and his wife had just arrived at the French Riviera to spend their vacation, they went to the beach. His wife went in the water for a while, then coated herself with sun-lotion and settled down to relax. Suddenly it struck Wayne that he was lying there in a lounge chair, halfway around the world from home, reading some books and papers he had brought from the office. For the first time in his life, he had to admit that he was hooked on working. He couldn't even leave it behind for a trip to the beach!

Wayne sent me an autographed copy of his book and signed it "from one workaholic to another."

I had to admit it was true — I was one too. But it had been a long time since I had taken my work to the beach. I had taken it on vacation, yes. But not to the beach.

As much as I liked to work — as much as it recharged my batteries — I also knew that working all the time makes us miss some very important things. Whatever we're doing in life, whether it's work or play or something in-between, diverts our attention from other things we might be doing.

We simply can't have it all and do it all at the same time. I have worked hard all my life and have loved doing it, but I know I've missed some things because of it.

I recently met a man named Mike who was a tax accountant most of his life. Since retiring, he has started writing haiku. He talked endlessly about his "haiku moments" — the unforgettable occasion when he saw a red sunrise over the geysers at Yellowstone or heard an owl calling in the woods behind his house or enjoyed the unique flavor of a cup of chai. These have become worth more to him, he said, than all his years of laboring over other people's books in order to earn a living. The morning I met him, he had seen a sparrow land on the top of a tall blade of grass, then ride it back and forth for a few minutes before flying away.

"I still shiver," he said, "when I think about it!"

Mike was right, of course. Work kept him from many such experiences. But, while I didn't say this to him, I wondered if there weren't haiku moments at work too, if he had only been looking for them.

That was one thing I tried to do when I was working so hard. I attempted not to miss any of the special moments of my day. Whenever one of my sons came into the study, I stopped what I was doing and gave him my full attention. I didn't miss many opportunities to hug my beautiful wife. As a teacher, I cherished my students, and tried to see the beauty and uniqueness in each of them. And in the churches I pastored I tried to be alert to all the holy things going on in people's lives — the way little old ladies put their lipstick on crooked, the way children couldn't stay in line when marching into the church sanctuary, the way some of the older men looked like angelic little boys when they put on their choir robes.

I'm sure I missed a lot. We can't concentrate on anything without missing something else. Right now, as I am writing this, my wife is preparing dinner and I am not as fully aware as I might be of the piquant smells wafting up from the kitchen, the little noises of preparation, the way she has bent over the candles at the table to remove the wax that dripped down their sides.

I accept missing things as part of the price of doing anything. We can't feel and respond to everything. If we were and did, we would probably die of paralysis, unable to breathe for fear we would miss something. Life is full of compromises and this is one of them.

I celebrate work — especially any work that doesn't diminish our sensibilities. Even accountants like Mike, I am sure, can live with awareness — and lab technicians and grocery clerks and auto mechanics.

Any kind of work is a gift. At my time of life I can look back and realize that my work is me — that whatever I have produced is somehow a lasting monument to who I am now. When I am gone it will live on as a testimony to my having come this way. I ponder the joy of people in other callings — the architect who walks among the buildings he has built, the doctor who remembers the people she has healed, the poet who can read his haiku moments in all the sonnets he has written, the gardener who remembers when he planted this or that tree, the moviemaker who can point to a series of films and say, "There, there is the evidence of my mind, my thinking, my interaction with the world!"

We are, in some ways, what we have done. It is a good feeling. It is an offering to God. It is part of what it means to be spiritual that we can recognize this when we have finished, and say, as J. S. Bach wrote on the manuscripts of many of his compositions, "S.D.G." — *soli deo gloria* — "To God alone be the glory!"

Six

The Don Quixote Factor

I don't think I have ever been a one-note person. I have always cared enormously about life in all its beauty and variety, and this in turn has led me to a lively interest in many things. I have been deeply devoted to the people in my family, my classes, and my congregations, as well as others I happened to meet along the way. And from the days of my early religious experiences I have felt a profound interest in human spirituality and how we can transcend our obvious limitations to live more consciously in the presence of God. I might point out also my enjoyment of such disparate activities as traveling, going to the theater, hiking, swimming, playing tennis, gardening, making things (my most ambitious projects were a toolshed and a roomful of cabinetry and book shelves), writing poetry, and drawing colorful posters for family birthdays. Friends have often called me a "renaissance man," though more in the spirit of bonhommie, I am sure, than of accuracy.

Yet there is, in spite of this, a single thing for which I shall probably be remembered by many people, and which I myself regard as an unintended natural consequence of who I am and how I have reacted to certain things I have encountered in life. That is my decades-long aversion to what I consider to be dishonesty in public religion and the kind of hypocrisy that inevitably arises from people's attempting to use religion for personal or corporate benefits. Naively, I suppose, I always regarded religion as holy, as sacrosanct, as belonging to God; and therefore anybody who traduced or perverted it was simply doing wrong.

I have never thought of myself as being prophetic, and did not start out to make the world over according to my own ways and desires. All of that simply happened, to the extent that I was at all prophetic or tried to remake anything, because I cared about some things and felt from time to time that it was my duty to speak out about them. If I ended up being some kind of Don Quixote, idealistically tilting at windmills, it wasn't intentional, it was simply in my nature to do that.

☙

To begin with, I am a very stubborn person. I don't mean to be. I actually think of myself as being very flexible, and usually try to see both sides of every question. On the Myers-Briggs Typology chart, I am clearly "perceptive" and not "judgmental," which means that I have very few strong feelings about what other people do because I can imagine all kinds of reasons for their doing it. While it is an admittedly objectionable example, I could probably even manufacture excuses for Adolph Hitler's becoming the kind of monster he was. But, along with this almost total flexibility and understanding, which my wife says can be very annoying at times, particularly when I cannot get angry at someone about whom she is fuming, I have a deep vein of determination and stubbornness in my character. One could almost say it is a mother-lode.

I don't know where it came from. Perhaps from my father and his family, who, once they formed an opinion about anything, seldom abandoned it. Certainly not from my mother's side of the family, for they were all as sweet and agreeable as a bowl of pudding. But my stubbornness, in one who is customarily so light-hearted and *laissez-faire*, is really my own, and I cannot blame it on anyone else.

It first came to light, when I was twelve years old, in a very interesting way.

I was walking home from school one afternoon with a boy named Herbert. Herbert was a lot older than I was, and a great deal larger. It may be only my imagination, but I now recall his standing some twelve or fifteen inches taller than I was. I liked Herbert. Even though he was one of the four or five boys in my class who had failed to be promoted several times and thus were not only older but also much bigger and stronger than the rest of us, he was not a bully, as most of them were. I didn't believe he was dumb. He had unfortunately got labeled as a failure in the system and was therefore destined to fulfill its prediction. I felt sorry for him.

That day was in fact Herbert's sixteenth birthday, and he had just announced it to me, together with the information that his mother was making him a birthday cake and had already said that he might drop out of school at the end of the current term and start earning a living. I could tell that he was happy about it, and I was happy for him.

So I slapped him on the back and said, "Congratulations, you lucky son of a bitch!"

I don't know why I said that. I didn't normally use that kind of language. In fact, I abhorred it, and I wasn't even sure what a son of a bitch was. My dad often used the term — usually in addressing me — but I wasn't really certain of its meaning. I think I just wanted to say something upbeat and congratulatory to Herbert and that phrase inadvertently came out of my mouth. I know I said it with a definite lilt and the best of intentions.

Herbert obviously knew what it meant — literally — and was unhappy with it. He said something about not insulting his mother, but I couldn't be exactly sure what he said because at the same time that he said it his fist was flying out and connecting with my face, so that it sent me flying onto the ground in somebody's yard that we were passing.

I should have got up and apologized and said, "I don't know why I said that. I don't even know what it means — or didn't until this minute. Please forgive me, Herbert."

But my sense of indignation was far stronger than any desire to apologize, so I stood up — wobblely, I'm sure — and called him a son of a bitch again.

Wham! He struck me again, sending me reeling into the *next* yard on the block.

Once more I climbed to my feet and hurled the epithet.

Wham! Herbert hit me again, and this time I decorated the *next* yard.

I think I went down in every yard for two blocks that afternoon, until we came to the corner where Herbert's home lay in one direction, straight ahead, and mine lay to the right, up Harvey's Hill and out into the country beyond. I turned to go up the hill, but I kept on yelling the words "son of a bitch" at him. I can still see Herbert standing there, bewildered about whether to pursue me and continue beating the stuffing out of me or to go on home to his mother and the birthday cake. Fortunately, home and mother and the cake won, and he eventually trudged on toward them.

Herbert did leave school in a few weeks and I didn't see him again for years. When I did see him, I was back home visiting my parents and pulled into a Shell station to fill up the car with gas. Herbert was working at the station. He had gone into military service, he said, had put in twenty years, and was now discharged and living on his pension.

We were happy to see one another and catch up on what we'd been doing. Neither of us mentioned the "son-of-a-bitch" episode. I still felt sorry for him.

And I still think about the episode. Why didn't I apologize and put an end to my suffering? Herbert was right to hit me. As he understood better than I did, I had insulted his mother. But that was the point, as I reflect on it. I was mad because I had not understood and had not meant to insult his mother. I had intended the offensive words as a congratulatory message, nothing more. So I perceived an injustice in Herbert's striking me. And that was why I could not let it go, why I had to keep bouncing back for more punishment.

My wife, Anne, told this story at my seventieth-birthday party. She had everybody in stitches about it. She told it, she said, because she thought it was revelatory of who I was and am. I have always had what she called my "s.o.b. determination." It explained a lot about me, she said — about the fact that I had earned not one but two doctorates, about all the books I'd written, about the unpopular stands I'd sometimes adopted as a pastor, and about the way I'd stood up to the fundamentalists when so few were doing it.

I'm sure she was right, because now I can see the dots in my life and how they connect. I can see the times when I thought an injustice was being done to somebody — it wasn't usually me — and I had to say so. I can see the times when I believed that religion was being used and misrepresented for some unworthy end and I couldn't remain quiet about it. I can remember some of the sermons I preached, and how they support my wife's contention. Dot by dot by dot, they all connect, and they lead to who I am now and what a lot of people identify as the real me.

৵

The Golden Gate Seminary affair was such a dot.

It was 1966, only a year after I went to teach at Vanderbilt Divinity School. I had been invited to address the annual Missions Conference at Golden Gate Baptist Theological Seminary in Mill Valley, California. There would be eight hundred college students present, and I was asked to speak to them on the subject "Christ in a World in Revolution." In accordance with the seminary's policy, I submitted my lectures to the administration several days before the conference.

Apparently somebody was asleep at the switch and didn't red-flag a few brief remarks in the second lecture, which I called "Christ *Is* a Revolution," about the lack of honesty and originality at the Southern Baptist Sunday School Board, which just happened to be the seminary's major source of funding. The Sunday School Board was in Nashville, where I lived. I knew a fair number of people who worked for the board. They were all intelligent, personable men and women, many of whom were imaginative and creative. But the things they thought and believed never made it out of the board's offices to the world beyond. Everything my friends said or wrote was bowdlerized and sanitized for public consumption, so that it wouldn't offend anyone. But that offended me, I said. I wanted my religion to be less generic and more particular, with a whiff of genuine human sweat and personality about it.

Immediately after I completed this lecture, which was given on a Sunday morning, the president of the seminary, Dr. Harold Graves, took the microphone to rebut what I had said and, if possible, to delete it from the students' minds. "We *are* free," he repeated with droning monotony for ten or fifteen minutes while one of his assistants confiscated printed copies of the address prepared for distribution to the students, as well as taped copies being recorded for the school's archives.

I was flabbergasted! I had never before encountered such anger and hostility toward anything I had said. I thought schools were places where thoughts and opinions could be aired. Later I learned that there had been a representative from the Sunday School Board in the meeting and that the seminary was coming up shortly for its annual appropriation. The president was in a bind and felt compelled to take action. The following day he played a tape of my address at a specially called faculty meeting and attempted to persuade the professors to sign a paper condemning it. Some of the wiser ones counseled moderation and a majority of others agreed.

Frustrated, Graves got in his car and sped off to Fresno, where he played the tape of my lecture for Dr. Terry Young, the editor of California's Southern Baptist newspaper. Young, who had political aspirations in the Southern Baptist Convention and later became a professor of theology at New Orleans Baptist Theological Seminary, wrote a scurrilous editorial accusing me not only of being a heretic but of being immoral. The basis of the latter charge was that I had used an illustration from James Baldwin's novel *Giovanni's Room*. Everybody knew Baldwin was a homosexual, so *ipso facto* I was immoral.

A few days later President Graves brought a tape of my lecture to the Southern Baptist Convention's executive board meeting in Nashville and played it there. While everybody was listening, he collapsed. At first it was thought that he had a heart attack. But doctors at the Baptist Hospital said he was merely suffering from nervous exhaustion and sent him home with orders to take a long vacation.

The executive secretary of the Sunday School Board, Dr. James L. Sullivan, a man I had always supposed to be fair and sensible, telephoned that same afternoon to ask if I would come to his office. I said I would be glad to and asked when he would like me to come. He said it must be right then, as he was leaving the next day for the Philippines. I said that was impossible, as my wife was out shopping and I was at home with a sick child. So Dr. Sullivan asked if he could come to our home. I knew that if he was going to fly halfway around the world the next day his visit must be extremely serious.

In less than thirty minutes he was at our front door. I led him into the den and offered him something to drink. He declined, saying he didn't have much time and wanted to get right down to business. He commenced attacking me for my "bad attitude" toward the Sunday School Board, which apparently had something to do with "recrucifying" Christ. For more than an hour he reproached me for what I had said in my lecture and how it would undermine people's confidence in the Sunday School Board. At one point he demanded that I attend a board meeting and see for myself how free its members were. I said I would be happy to do that, but only on the condition that I could bring along some acquaintances who were no longer at the board and would be able to verify whether I was seeing a typical meeting or one rigged to create a special impression. Still fuming, Sullivan finally left and drove away, presumably to finish packing for his trip to the Philippines.

A few weeks later, advertisements appeared for that summer's Sunday School Board camp weeks at Ridge Crest, North Carolina, and Glorieta, New Mexico. I had been scheduled for lectures at both meetings and Anne and I had looked forward to going. But now my name was conspicuously missing from the programs. I telephoned an official at the board. It was true, he said, my name did not appear on the lists of speakers. I requested an official notification that my name had been intentionally dropped. He said he could not give me one. I had simply become *persona non grata* in the Southern Baptist Convention.

For years, the scandal of Golden Gate dogged me wherever I went, especially among Baptists. Once, the Baptist student minister at Berea College in Kentucky phoned to ask why I had given in to the board.

"What are you talking about?" I asked.

He said that a vice president from Golden Gate Seminary had been on the Berea campus recruiting students, and in a public gathering one of the students had challenged him by asking, "What about the Killinger affair?" Without batting an eye the vice president replied, "That is all behind us now. Dr. Sullivan and the Executive Board gave a dinner with Dr. Killinger as their guest. Dr. Sullivan made a speech in which he openly forgave Dr. Killinger, and Dr. Killinger wept and they embraced."

I was really devastated by all of this. I had always been a Baptist and had never considered joining another church, even when friends at Harvard and Princeton were playing musical chairs with denominations in order to go where they could find the best venues for their talents. Now my own denomination had rejected me, at least at the official level. The worst part was that we lived in Nashville, where Southern Baptists' headquarters were. Many people who had been our friends and worked at the Sunday School Board would not speak to us, even in the church where we were members. One of our oldest and dearest friends at the board, Howard Bramlette, on more than one occasion walked across the street only yards ahead of us in order to avoid speaking.

Years later Howard apologized. "The word at the board," he said, "was that anybody seen speaking to you would be fired."

Dismissal was obviously the board's method of controlling people. I said I appreciated Vanderbilt's reaction to my problem. A few days after I stepped on the land mine at Golden Gate Seminary — before President Graves brought the tapes to the executive board meeting — Dr. Sullivan telephoned Vice Chancellor Rob Roy Purdy at Vanderbilt, described the trouble I had made for the board, and asked Purdy to release me from my teaching position.

"That may be the way you run the Sunday School Board," responded Purdy drily, "but it isn't the way we treat faculty members at Vanderbilt."

I still have many dear friends who are ministers of Southern Baptist churches, and I sympathize with them for the fine line they have to walk in order to preserve their right to serve where they do. But it was clear, after the debacle at Golden Gate Seminary, that my own career as a Southern Baptist clergyman was over. The ramifications of those few seconds' worth of monologue about Jesus as a revolutionary and an anti-institutionalist have spread like ripples on a pond over my entire life and career, eroding my desire to serve the denomination I grew up in and setting me loose in the religious world as an essentially free agent. But it is hard to have an independent perspective in an institution as basically conservative as the church without appearing to be radical.

I could have capitulated, of course, and issued a statement apologizing for my "ill-considered" remarks about the Sunday School Board. Few people would ever have noticed the turn-around, or cared, even if they had noticed. But my friends would have noticed — especially those I had made on the faculty at Golden Gate Seminary — and I would have been ashamed before them. And even more importantly, I would have been ashamed before my own conscience. My "s.o.b. determination" wouldn't let me do it.

My next really big s.o.b. moment came when I went to Lynchburg, Virginia, as minister of the First Presbyterian Church. I went to Lynchburg with the single intention of being the best minister I could. I was putting my academic life behind and moving on to be a minister in the trenches. I had no idea I would end up locking horns with the Rev. Mr. Jerry Falwell and becoming an outspoken lifelong opponent of the kind of narrow, fundamentalist religion he espoused.

It began when I preached a sermon called "Would Jesus Appear on the Old-Time Gospel Hour?" I honestly had no intention of using the sermon to attack Falwell and his widely televised program. I only meant to use an imaginary confrontation between Jesus and the OTGH as an opener for questioning the religion of our own congregation. I posed the question about Jesus and then said, in effect, "Yes, Jesus would probably appear on the program. He often accepted such challenges. But he would ask his host some embarrassing questions about what they do with all the money they take in and why they don't show a greater concern for the poor."

Then, having gotten my congregation's rapt attention, I said as casually as I could, "We ourselves could not expect very polite talk from Jesus if he were here this morning. We would be no more exempt from his laserlike wrath or stinging comments than the cherubic-faced performers of 'The Old-Time Gospel Hour.'" And I proceeded to list some of the indictments Jesus might level against us: that our pride in our elegant sanctuary and beautiful stained-glass windows would not save us from the judgment to come; that we spent far too much time preparing our faces and bodies for church and far too little preparing our souls before God; that the poor of the world would rise up and condemn us for caring more about our hymns and creeds and sacraments than we did about compassion and justice for the neglected peoples of the world.

But in the Lynchburg of the eighties nobody heard what I was saying about our own church. They were too shocked that anybody living in the community would dare to question Jerry Falwell and his empire. He was, as the Chamber of Commerce was fond of pointing out, the third largest employer in the county, just behind General Electric and Babcock-Wilcox, the nuclear power company. He was hands-down the town's most famous citizen. The residents of Lynchburg held more of his church bonds — already condemned by a federal judge for fraudulence — than the stocks and bonds of any other company. The only local newspaper idolized him. President Reagan appeared publicly with him. He was a celebrity. In the eyes of many, he was clearly God's anointed.

Lynchburg was a close-knit community. It was also a drinking town. There were few afternoons when somebody didn't throw a big cocktail party somewhere. And the hot topic of conversation at all the cocktail hours that week was what the minister at First Presbyterian Church had said about Jerry Falwell. I felt the way Martin Luther said he felt when he nailed the Ninety-five Theses to the door of the Wittenberg Cathedral — as if he had been sleepwalking, had seized the church's bell rope, and had inadvertently awakened the whole town!

Thus began five years of verbal combat between Jerry and me. The next Sunday on his radio program he said, "We don't need Dr. Killinger in this town. Now, I don't want any of you to do anything to hurt him, but we certainly don't want him here. We have a lot of friends in First Presbyterian Church. I know they're ashamed of their pastor and would like him to leave. Some of them have told me so this week. He doesn't belong in this town."

Strange things began to happen. My children received phone calls warning that their father was going to die. Our garbage was picked up in the night after we set it at the curb, before the regular truck came to collect it. Our phones were tapped. Once, a U.S. Post Office inspector called to say that somebody had reported a batch of mail burning on Liberty Mountain, where Falwell's property was located, and it was addressed to me. I spoke with the inspector several times. Then he suddenly disappeared and the postal service wouldn't tell me how to get in touch with him, even though I phoned them repeatedly. For three years the IRS audited our tax returns with a fine-toothed comb — until I told some reporters in Murfreesboro, Tennessee, that it was happening and they wrote an article about it. Then it stopped as mysteriously as it had begun.

Falwell did have supporters in my church. Several of them. And all of them were either wealthy or well connected. They were uncomfortable with my taking sides against their man in the media. And the media were everywhere, once it got out that one of Falwell's fellow clergymen was speaking freely about him. I was featured in *People* magazine. Douglas Kiker brought an NBC News team to Lynchburg and interviewed me standing in front of our beautiful sanctuary building. David Frost sent a brace of reporters from London, who said they would ask me the questions and then Frost's picture and voice would be patched in for the final editing. Dozens of journalists interviewed me for books they were writing. And it made my church members very nervous. After all, some of them were heavily invested in Falwell's future.

I didn't want to make a nuisance of myself on the religious scene. All I really wanted to do was to be a good pastor and take care of my own flock. But once you take a stand on a public issue, the way I did over Falwell, you can't easily walk away from it. It's like holding onto a fire hose when somebody turns the water on — you can't let go of it then even if you want to. And besides, I began to think that maybe standing up to Falwell was the reason I had been led to Lynchburg.

Maybe I shouldn't have gone on criticizing Falwell. Having seen what a ruckus I was causing, perhaps I should have let it all drop. But I was honestly fearful of where the combination of fundamentalist religion and right-wing politics was going to lead us. Professor Eberhard Bethje, the son-in-law of Dietrich Bonhoeffer, spent several semesters lecturing at Lynchburg College, a Disciples of Christ institution, during the early 1980s, and ominously declared that he could see the same collusion between religion and government in this country that he had witnessed in Nazi Germany in the 1930s. We haven't reached that point yet, but there are signs that we may be even closer to it now than we were during my Lynchburg years.

I tried to be a good pastor in spite of the energy it took to carry on the anti-Falwell fight. My concerns about fundamentalism never interfered with my duties as a minister. I always used sermons as a way to clarify the meaning of the Gospel for people in the twentieth century, and as a result I was able to minimalize the criticisms of my public stance among my own congregants. Even when I preached a sermon about fundamentalism's distorted view of things, which I did perhaps once every six months, it was invariably a sermon aimed at helping my own people to find their way in a maze of ethical and religious options.

⌒⌒

Our last year in Lynchburg, one of Falwell's friends who was a member of our congregation at First Presbyterian came to me and said, "Some of us think it's a pity that you and Rev. Falwell have been dueling with one another all this time and don't really know one another personally. We'd like to propose that you and he meet once a month for lunch or dinner and become better acquainted. Would you be willing?"

I didn't have to think long, as I didn't believe that Falwell would welcome the chance to spend time with me.

"Sure," I said. "Falwell's probably the most interesting man in town."

"Fine," said the man, "Falwell has already agreed!"

I made the first overture, and set up lunch at a neutral restaurant. Then Anne and I had Jerry and his wife, Macel, to our home for dinner. It was an interesting evening, and we enjoyed it, although it was clear that Falwell was very uneasy when the conversation got around to anything religious or theological. Then he became very formal, as if reading a script off the inside of his forehead, and changed the subject.

During this time, Falwell and I were both scheduled to be speakers at a series of community Lenten services sponsored by the ministerial association and held at a downtown Episcopalian church. As Falwell was the first speaker in the series and I the last, Anne and I went to hear what he had to say. All the speakers scheduled for the series were asked to deal with the biblical subject of peace, but he didn't mention it once. His sermon was devoted entirely to the subject of salvation.

After the service, which was held just before lunch, Falwell came down out of the chancel, waved at us, and hollered with a volume that could be easily heard anywhere in the sanctuary, "John! Anne! Come go to England with me!" He was flourishing a fistful of first-class airline tickets that the White House had just sent him to fly to England and debate with

Prime Minister Robert Menzies of New Zealand at the Oxford English-Speaking Club. The subject of discussion was to be the deployment of nuclear forces in NATO. The White House said he could take along anybody he liked.

"Jerry," I asked, "what do you know about nuclear forces and NATO?"

"Nothing," he cheerfully admitted. "But they'll brief me on the way over."

In those days, Falwell liked to brag that he could enter the Oval Office on five minutes' notice. I never saw any evidence to contradict such a claim. He had enormous influence on Ronald Reagan, even though I think Reagan was secretly wary of him and the fundamentalists. Almost every week, I was told, he flew members of Congress or the president's cabinet to Lynchburg to speak at Liberty University's chapel service, gave them a check for ten thousand dollars from OTGH funds, and had them back in Washington for lunch. To his credit, Reagan never came to Lynchburg to adorn Falwell's program, but Vice President George H. W. Bush did.

℃੭

When we left Lynchburg after six years, I breathed a sigh of relief, thinking my struggle with the fundamentalists was over. We had barely landed in Los Angeles, however, when I had a phone call from the Michael Jackson Show asking if I would appear for a discussion with Michael about the fundamentalist phenomenon in America. This Michael Jackson was from South Africa, and for years had emceed a popular national radio show. Now he was piloting a new TV show as well, and it was to this show that I was invited.

I had no idea Michael was setting me up. Jerry Falwell was in Anaheim that week to speak to a conference of conservative Christian educators. He was scheduled to be on Michael's program the next day. When Falwell came on, Michael introduced him, then began showing clips of what I had said the day before and asking Falwell to comment on my remarks.

"Oh, John Killinger had a nervous breakdown in Lynchburg," Falwell said glibly. "He had to leave his church. His own church members didn't want him any more. He had to go."

Someone phoned Anne and told her to turn on the TV set. She did, and cried at the outrageous things Falwell was saying as if they were completely true. Later, she wrote him a five-page letter telling him exactly what she thought about him and what he had done. She said she felt entitled to write him because he had mentioned her on the program. While he was vilifying me, he said, "But his wife's great! She's a beautiful woman! I know Anne's ashamed of her husband." We never heard from Rev. Falwell again.

❧

Not personally and directly, that is. But our feud wasn't over.

In 1989, as I have said, I left Los Angeles to become a professor at Samford University. As Samford's first university professor — one entitled to teach any subject in any department — I went with the understanding that my office would be in the new Beeson Divinity School. Even though I taught in the English and religion departments as well, I was well known as a teacher of preaching and expected to do most of my work with graduate students in the divinity school.

The money to found Beeson Divinity School was given to Samford by Ralph Waldo Beeson, a retired insurance executive who had made his fortune with the Liberty Mutual Insurance Company in Birmingham, Alabama. Beeson was a member of the Independent Presbyterian Church, a dignified old institution in a once-proud area of the city. His wife, who was deceased, had been a United Methodist. So as Beeson began disposing of his wealth, he gave equal amounts to Asbury Theological Seminary in Asbury, Kentucky, a conservative Methodist school that his wife admired, and Samford University, which, although it was a Baptist school, lay in the valley below his home where he could "keep watch on it from above."

One of Beeson's primary stipulations for the new divinity school was that it should be thoroughly ecumenical and not merely a replica of other

Baptist seminaries. Accordingly, he specified that there must be at least six faculty chairs for distinguished non-Baptist scholars. Beeson's "chaplain" at Independent Presbyterian Church, an older minister named Fred Widmer, was already serving part-time on the new divinity faculty as professor of pastoral care. As a Congregationalist, I was the second non-Baptist appointment. Gerald Bray, an Anglican church history professor from Cambridge University, was the third. But the dean of the school, selected a year before I arrived on the scene, was a Southern Baptist named Timothy George, who, following Beeson's death and the school's receipt of the fifty-million-dollar bequest, made little effort to attract non-Baptists, especially any who might be distinguished enough to raise a voice against his own designs and policies for the school.

I did not realize how bitterly George opposed my appointment. He was a competent scholar. He had taken his doctorate at Harvard with George Huntston Williams, one of my favorite professors there, and then had taught church history for several years at Southern Baptist Theological Seminary in Louisville. I assumed that he was a reasonable choice to head up the new school. But he had developed a strong interest in the work of the sixteenth-century theologian John Calvin, and, calling himself a Calvinist, forged strong connections with the fundamentalist movement that was in the process of taking over the Southern Baptist Convention. I did not know at the time when I went to Samford that George also had an extremely friendly relationship with Jerry Falwell.

I tried to be tolerant of George's right-wing brand of Christianity, because I respected his intelligence and honestly believed that Christians should be able to be friends even though they differ widely on points of theological understanding. George and I occasionally lunched together during my first two years at Samford, and talked openly about our differences. At least, *I* talked about them.

The interesting thing about us, I said, was that my pilgrimage had made me more open to other points of view, while his had made him more closed. I remember suggesting once that his religious views made him very centripetal; he wanted to find God at the very center of his system and tended to repudiate anything not oriented toward that center. My views, on the other hand, made me centrifugal; I expected to find God in the universe beyond my own and thus wanted to embrace everything as holy. He wanted everything *reduced* to God; I wanted everything *expanded* to God. I still think that succinctly defines the difference between us.

What it came down to was that George was very authoritarian, both as a theologian and as an administrator. If he believed something to be true, there was no room in his system for anything else to be true. He had obviously never had the kind of experience I had had that afternoon in Paris when I went to the Arrabal play and came out of the theater with the sense that the cacophony and uproar inside were more real than the peaceful streets outside. If he disagreed with a position, whether it was teleological or theological, he simply dismissed it as having no foundation whatsoever.

Consequently, like Falwell, George wasn't a collegial administrator. He liked to deliver his mandates without extending the possibility of discussion. At my first divinity-school faculty meeting I asked for the reasons behind certain decisions being announced. Afterward, George informed me that I wasn't really meant to attend divinity faculty meetings, because I was a university professor and therefore not actually part of his school.

He did everything he could to discourage my participation in the divinity school. During my first year he excluded me from teaching the required preaching and worship courses I had believed I would be offering by saying he had assigned those to someone else before he knew I was coming. Then, when I gave him a list of titles and descriptions for the courses I wished to offer the second year, he said dismissively that he liked the way the other professor was teaching them and intended for him to continue. The other professor was not qualified to teach them, but the dean liked him because he was an unquestioning fundamentalist.

At that time there were about a hundred students in the entire divinity school, and most of them, because of a heavy schedule of graduation requirements, were forced to take required courses. Therefore my courses, all electives, were disappointingly small. Later I learned from some of the students that they had been systematically warned not to enroll in my courses lest I lead them into theological error. I also learned that George was complaining to the provost that my enrollments were too small to justify my participation in the divinity school, and suggesting that I be restricted to teaching in the English and undergraduate religion departments, where I was also offering courses.

Disillusioned, I tried to soldier on, deriving what pleasure I could from my writing and off-campus preaching and lecturing. In December of 1992, Anne and I flew to England to commence a one-semester sabbatical at Oxford. Soon I forgot the tensions at Samford and immersed myself in two or three writing projects, including a book on Zen Buddhism. When we flew home the following summer, we arrived at the Birmingham airport a little after midnight and were amazed to find a large number of friends, including two professors and a secretary from the divinity school, waiting to greet us. But they knew something we didn't know. They had known it, in fact, for several months.

While we were in England, Jerry Falwell had visited the campus as a guest of the Cumberland School of Law. During an open forum, a Samford student had asked Falwell what he thought about me. Falwell delivered a blustering tirade about me and said that I ought not to be allowed to teach in a Christian school like Samford.

I do not know if Timothy George took his cue from that public statement by Falwell or if he and Falwell met privately and Falwell pressed him to do so, but shortly after the Falwell visit George ordered all my courses and course descriptions canceled from the divinity school computers. The friends who appeared at the airport that night knew it had been done, and were trying to demonstrate their support, even though not one of them uttered a word about what had happened.

When I learned the truth from a secretary in the divinity school, I went directly to the president's office. He was out of town. So I went to the provost's office, and demanded to know why I had not been told of George's action. The provost admitted that he and the president had acquiesced in the dean's decision because they thought it "would be best for the school." When I asked why he had not called me to talk about it, he said that he had intended to but had not got around to it. Then he said, "Actually, I thought it was the sort of thing we should talk about in person."

My academic life — indeed, my professional life as a whole, as I was now sixty years old — was essentially shattered. I said as much to President Corts when we had lunch later in the summer, but he merely shrugged his shoulders and said I was still free to teach in other parts of the university. I think he honestly did not understand, because he had never had an academic subject area to which he devoted his life and work, the integral relationship between a professor's spirit and the particular area of his or her expertise. He might as earnestly have counseled Einstein to be happy with an appointment in the chemistry department or Stephen Sondheim to be satisfied with staging the plays of Shakespeare.

Because I still had to earn a living, I remained at Samford for four more years, teaching in the English and religion departments. When the divinity school moved into its posh new building, I was left behind to occupy an old office that hadn't been redecorated since World War II. Paint had peeled off the gray walls and the ancient carpet was so faded and stained that it was hard to tell what color it really was. On the wall behind my desk hung an old painting of the biblical scapegoat — the animal that was driven into the wilderness after the high priest had performed his annual ritual of laying the sins of the people on it. I felt related to that goat and often had conversations with it. I would have liked to take the painting with me when we left Birmingham, but didn't want anyone to accuse me of stealing university property.

⌒

Looking back now, I realize that there were probably a number of points at which I might have ameliorated my situation by weeping, begging, promising to be less openly heretical, or generally eating crow. Institutions seldom care what people are like in the inner sanctums of their own hearts and minds. They are only interested in conformity and the ability to get on with their agendas without having to stop and fuss over the people in their employ. But I had too much s.o.b. determination to turn aside from my own gifts, ideas, and mission for the sake of an uneasy peace. I could never, had I been Galileo, have recanted my discovery that the sun, not the earth, was the center of the solar system. I am sure I would have gone to the stake in the fierce knowledge that someday people would understand what I already understood and condemn the barbarians who took my life.

I conferred with some attorneys to see if I could compel the university to honor our original agreement and permit me to teach in the divinity school. They were thoughtful, reasonable men and I soon developed an enormous respect for them. I knew they believed in the rightness of my cause because they offered to pursue the case on a contingency basis. Following their advice, I initiated legal action and felt hopeful, if not confident, that justice would be served. After months of depositions, conferences, memos, briefs, and waiting — always waiting — a federal judge in Birmingham decided that the court could not find against a religious institution on a matter involving a professor who alleged discriminatory behavior because of theological differences.

My attorneys appealed to the Eighth Judicial Circuit Court in Atlanta. There the same judges who a short time later would find against Albert Gore in the matter of the 2000 presidential election in Florida ruled three-to-nothing against us. Given the makeup of the Supreme Court, which would uphold the decision against Gore, my attorneys decided that it would be imprudent and even futile to appeal to that body. As far as they were concerned, the fight was over. They would have a hard time, they said, getting their law firm to support a continued struggle.

One by one, as the litigation had dragged on, my friends at Samford had fallen away. I felt like a virtual outcast among the faculty — like the goat on my wall — because I was challenging the authority of the institution that paid their salaries. Eventually, as I became more and more of a pariah, it seemed sensible to leave. That was when I decided to spend all my summers at Mackinac Island and wrote to President Corts saying I had been disappointed in my experience at Samford and thought it was time to sever our relationship. President Corts never responded.

ᖍᖑ

Anne was right, I did grow up with a lot of s.o.b. determination. And that determination, I now see clearly, marked the significant trajectory of my life. There were certain things I simply had to do and couldn't back away from. I might have had a softer, easier time of it if I had been more flexible or malleable. But that wasn't who I was.

Maybe I do have a Don Quixote complex. I know that I never feel more certain of who I am or where the truth lies than when I'm tilting at some windmill that is likely to knock me off my horse and leave me flat on my back, the way Herbert did all those years ago. At least then I know that I'm not supporting a person or a cause because of anything it will do for me. I can be sure that my motives are purely altruistic.

Years ago, I read a story in *The Atlantic* about a Western ranch that had a phenomenal little burro they employed to break difficult steers. If a steer was unruly, they simply attached it to the burro by a short leash and turned the two out of the corral. The steer, larger and stronger, would toss the burro up and down as if it were weightless. They would disappear over the horizon, the poor burro alternately flying up in the air and being dragged behind the steer. But a few days later they would return very differently. The burro would be trotting in the lead and the steer would be following compliantly behind. It always happened that way. The burro's quiet persistence and ability to absorb punishment invariably won out over the massive strength of the steer.

I would like to think that I have made a difference in a lot of things by being stubbornly persistent like that little burro. But I know in all honesty that I haven't. In my case, the steer has won — again and again. Now, after years of battling fundamentalism and other forms of false religion, I realize that they are more rampant than ever, and growing stronger by the hour. I can hardly bear to look upon the contemporary religious scene in America. Love and tolerance and compassion have given way to hate and bigotry. Everything that was once mystical and transcendent and mythopoetic has been prostituted to greed and politics and self-promotion. I wouldn't find it at all surprising, while watching a TV news program, to see an ad with Paris Hilton promoting books about the rapture. It is all too much for me!

I hope God understands. If I have been wrong about everything, I'm sorry. If I have been ridiculous, tilting against insuperable odds and historical inevitabilities, then I humbly apologize. But I have merely been who I was, honestly and truly. I don't think I ever cut the cloth to favor the tailor. I only wanted to do what was right, and to do it in spite of the odds.

I don't believe it was an ego-trip. I'm sure I have a sound ego, but I don't think it was ever calculating or self-serving. I only wanted to be true to myself — Emerson was right about the heart vibrating to an iron string — and to the principles of Christ. And if there is one image that has encouraged me in all the truly decisive moments of my life, especially those involving taking a stand for everything that matters against everything that doesn't, it is the picture of Christ on the Cross, gritting his teeth and enduring the pain, not because he was saving the world, but because it was the right thing to do.

Now, reexamining my life and seeing all its work and play and commitment coming together like the strands of a beautiful, golden rope, I sometimes feel as if this particular bit — the Don Quixote thing — is the one knot that's hard to work into the whole. It's so unlike the rest of me, that is soft and relaxed and great on conflict-avoidance. In that respect, it seems like an alien part of my life, a big, fat scar that runs the whole length of it but isn't integral with the other parts. Still, I am happy to offer everything to God — including my s.o.b. determination — and let him be my judge.

A friend recently sent me this little prayer from the pen of Thomas Merton, and I affix it here because I completely agree with its sentiments: "My Lord God, I have no idea where I am going. I do not see the road ahead of me. I cannot know for certain where it will end. Nor do I really know myself, and the fact that I think that I am following your will does not mean that I am actually doing so. But I believe that the desire to please you does in fact please you. And I hope I have that desire in all that I am doing. I hope that I will never do anything apart from that desire. And I know that if I do this you will lead me by the right road though I may know nothing about it."

Seven

My Body, My Friend

Maybe it seems out of place to talk about the body in a book about spiritual life, but in my experience it is impossible to consider the spirit without it. The body is such a fantastic miracle, and so involved in how we feel, who we are, what we do with our lives, and how we relate to one another, that it cannot be omitted. I find that the older I become, the more attention I pay to mine. Not just because it breaks down more frequently — like an automobile with a lot of miles on it — but because it is such a wonder.

This morning I heard Diane Rehm interviewing Stephen Burns, who has recently published a book about Martin Luther King Jr. called *To the Mountaintop*. Early in the interview, Burns said that he saw King when he himself was only twelve years old, and knew when he looked in King's eyes that he was a holy man. For him, that single impression always overrode all others.

Someone phoned in to protest. "How can you say that a man who was a notorious womanizer was holy?" a woman's voice demanded.

I wanted to field the question myself. Burns said that King was always quite aware of the flaws in his makeup, and felt guilty about them. But I wouldn't have answered that way. I would have talked about how many religions of the world see a direct relation between sex and holiness, and would question whether one could really be holy unless one were also sexually aware and at home with his or her body.

We Christians may be far too hung up on sex, the way I suspect St. Paul was. He was always talking about the *sarx* and the *psuche,* the flesh and the spirit, as if they were polar opposites. But Jesus, I don't doubt, knew better. Flesh and spirit are really two rambunctious twins joined together for life.

From the moment we are born, we are sexual beings, longing to suck, touch, feel, and to be touched and fondled by others. We may discipline ourselves as we grow older, and learn appropriate times and manners for displaying our body-consciousness, but the older we become the more we realize that our personal history is one of bodily functions as much as it is of rational development and spirituality. And the two are so intertwined as to be literally inseparable, however much we have been taught by our prudish theology to deny it.

What did Sam Keen write way back there in *To a Dancing God* about getting up on one morning on the California coast and sitting there lazily with the sun on his back, that he wanted a theology that dealt with the body and didn't reject it outright because it was the body and therefore beneath discussion? Well, Sam was right. Christian theology has always been remiss for not dealing more positively with the physical side of life.

One of my very first memories of the consciousness of sex — or of my body — is of a time when I was a child of two or three and a doctor came to our house because I was ill. I don't know if the illness in any way involved the sexual organs, but I recall the doctor, a fat, youngish man who resembled Kilwilly on *Monarch of the Glen,* casually kneading my testicles and assuring my parents that I would be all right. Even at that age, I was embarrassed to be touched so intimately. He was, after all, a stranger, and I had not given my consent.

How did I know to resent his liberties? I cannot answer that. But I know that I did.

And the very first dream I can remember as a child is one from my first year of school. It was a sexual dream about my music teacher, who was younger and prettier than the other teachers. She was tied up in a chair, like the damsels in cowboy movies, and was completely helpless. She was also completely naked. I rescued her from her predicament and felt very protective of her. But the dream must also have embarrassed me, else why do I remember it as the very first dream I could recall? For a long time, I felt guilty about having had it.

Is the body thus bound to feelings of guilt? I can't recall anything my parents taught me, or anyone else, for that matter, that would have led me to believe so. Yet I did feel guilty about the dream. Maybe that is why St. Paul was so insistent on the evil of the flesh — because he felt guilty too, and believed that Christ somehow freed him from the consequences of his sins. This would go far toward explaining Christianity's success as a religion of guilt, particularly among Catholics and Puritans. And why the fundamentalists were so disturbed by Martin Scorcese's film *The Last Temptation of Christ,* in which Jesus on the Cross had erotic fantasies about Mary Magdalene. And why there has been such a hullabaloo about Dan Brown's novel *The Da Vinci Code,* which turns on Jesus' having been married to Mary Magdalene and her fleeing to France to bear his child.

It would also explain why most churches realize that the best time to recruit young people is during puberty, when their hormones are changing and they feel guilty about their nascent sexual desires.

❧

I bought all that stuff about religion and the body when I was young. Lust and damnation — masturbation and hellfire — self-flagellation for the sake of Christ — denying the power of the flesh — seeking a higher way — starving the body for the sake of the soul. Actually, I think, it made youth and sex an even more potent cocktail, so that the imagination constantly exploded into forbidden desire.

Literature was my salvation, I think. Especially D. H. Lawrence, who pointed to a deeper, more worldly-wise vision of sex and sensuality. I still relish that marvelous passage at the opening of his novel *The Rainbow,* about the Brangwen family's life on the farm and how intimately they were related to the earth: "They felt the rush of the sap in spring, they knew the wave which cannot halt, but every year throws forward the seed to begetting, and, falling back leaves the young-born on the earth. They knew the intercourse between heaven and earth, sunshine drawn into the breast and bowels, the rain sucked up in the daytime, nakedness that comes under the wind in autumn, showing the birds' nests no longer worth hiding. Their life and interrelations were such; feeling the pulse and body of the soil, that opened to their furrow for the grain, and became smooth and supple after their ploughing, and clung to their feet with a weight that pulled like desire, lying hard and unresponsive, when the crops were to be shorn away. The young corn waved and was silken, and the lustre slid along the limbs of the men who saw it. They took the udder of the cows, the cows yielded milk and pulse against the hands of the men, the pulse of the blood of the teats of the cows beat into the pulse of the hands of the men. They mounted their horses, and held life between the grip of their knees, they harnessed their horses at the wagon, and, with hand on the bridle-rings, drew the heaving of the horses after their will."[2]

After many years of reading both poetry and fiction, I know of no passage that so evokes my sense of the dance of life, the interchange of body and spirit, that is going on constantly on this little planet, whether or not one has the sensibility to see and feel it. And I put over against the suppleness of this prose, its lugubrious viscosity teeming with life, the figure of Paul Valéry's Monsieur Teste, in the little novel by that name, who is the consummate man of intelligence, devoted to eliminating passion in favor of mere thought. Teste, whose name is cognate with the French word *tête*, for "head," has spent his entire life in devotion to thinking and reflection, as opposed to acting and enjoying. His whole business is regulation, not participation, and his sole interest is in considering things, not feeling them. Every morning he sits and writes down what he is feeling as the sun rises. He reminds me of a saying by H. H. Farmer, that he was very suspicious of anybody who was always feeling his pulse to see how he felt about a sunset.

There is an innate health in the Brangwen family that is missing in M. Teste. Teste, in my opinion, is pathologically ill. The soul and spirit of human beings is vitally linked to body, earth, universe. To miss that connection is to miss everything. It is to be inhuman.

As a young country pastor, I sensed the common wholeness of the people in my little parishes, over against the general fever of the world. Most of them had scant education. Yet they knew the land, the copses, the cattle, sheep, and horses. They gave everything they had to the soil, and took back from it as they needed. They were generous to a fault, for they knew that all life is a gift from God, and a gift to be shared, not hoarded. In the summer they brought us sacks of vegetables from their gardens, and in the fall, packages of tenderloin from their slaughtering. They spoke with simple elegance, often mangling syntax to make sense. The very seasons took root in their lives and imparted a rhythm to them, as if they were little boats riding the tides of the year. They knew how to love and make love — not only among themselves but with the fields and the woods and the beasts that roamed in them.

Because I had lived among these people I felt more whole and sensible. Even though I spent much of my life in academic circles, I resisted becoming an intellectual, and strove instead to be a complete person, loving and laughing and enjoying my role as husband and parent. Today, looking back at what some might call my "achievements," I have little regard for the advanced degrees, the scholarly books and articles, the dog-tags of academia, and far more for the friends I made among my students, the years my family and I spent abroad on sabbaticals, the memories of playing ball with my children and making love to my wife.

Once, in a book called *The Fragile Presence: Transcendence in Modern Literature,* I commented on what I discerned as the spiritual dimensions of Henry Miller's "scandalous" prose in *Tropic of Cancer, Tropic of Capricorn,* and other books. Someone in Europe read it and gave a copy to Miller. He wrote me and said that I alone of all his critics had truly understood him, that there is a vapor of holiness about everything he ever did, because he sensed the presence of God in every act he ever performed, in the yearning and completion of every sexual liaison, and in all his writings about sex and the body electric. We carried on a correspondence for several years, and I treasure his letters. Miller lived intimately with the world, withholding nothing, revealing everything.

I still resonate to this passage from his book *The Wisdom of the Heart:* "I find that there is plenty of room in the world for everybody — great interspatial depths, great ego universes, great islands of repair, for whoever attains to individuality. On the surface, where the historical battles rage, where everything is interpreted in terms of money and power, there may be crowding but life only begins when one drops below the surface, when one gives up the struggle, sinks and disappears from sight. Now I can as easily not write as write: there is no longer any compulsion, no longer any therapeutic aspect to it. Whatever I do is done out of sheer joy: I drop my fruits like a ripe tree. What the general reader or the critic makes of it is not my concern. I am not establishing values: I defecate and nourish. There is nothing more to it."[3]

That is Miller the old man speaking, Miller the resident of Big Sur, sleeping when he felt like sleeping, rising when he felt like rising, eating when he was hungry and defecating when he had eaten. It is Miller the old warrior, Miller the monk who retreated from the world in order to embrace it, Miller the sage, the aged wise man who stared across the shining waves of the Pacific and felt the breezes of the centuries caressing his tanned, wrinkled body.

I know what he means — know it even better now than I did as a young man when I read *The Wisdom of the Heart.* I too am dropping my fruits like a ripe tree. I am not establishing values. There is something wonderful about age. We are never closer to God.

༄

I find it hard to think about my body without remembering my parents who created it. Their genes are in me. We are bound together forever, my ancestors and me, with all those who come after us. I looked recently on the face of our first grandchild, a little girl named Ellie Rose, who looks like her dad, who in turn they say looks like me. The imprint of generations is upon her, and in time she will probably pass it on to others.

My father, like his father before him, was tall and slender and handsome. Hollywood handsome, when he was young and his metabolism had not become a curse. Growing up on a farm, he always enjoyed hard physical labor. A cousin who used to watch him pitching hay on my maternal grandparents' farm said he had never seen a man as strong as my dad. Even in his seventies, he was still plowing and planting a huge garden, more than an acre of ground, and keeping it as clean and tidy as a finicky woman's parlor. He loved to perspire from working, and always said, if he had a cold or a fever, that it was the only way to cure it.

My mother was as soft and pretty as my father was hard and handsome. Looking at her youthful photographs, I can understand how my father fell in love with her. She too was strong and athletic, and loved to run. She was on the state girls' basketball team in Kentucky before many women engaged in popular sports, and could hit the basket four times out of five when hurling it overhand from the middle of the floor. One of my earliest memories of her, apart from the usual mother-and-child ones, is of seeing her riding a donkey in a donkey-basketball game, where the donkeys were shod in diapers and the gymnasium was full of people from our little town cheering for the teams.

At Farm Bureau picnics, which we always attended because my father was a county agricultural agent, she always won the women's foot race, running barefoot because that was the way she had grown up running on the farm. And it was a disappointment if the man who won the men's race in a particular year didn't challenge her to race with him. When he did, she invariably won that as well.

I am glad to have the bodies of those two people represented now in my own flesh. I fancy I inherited my father's strength and my mother's swiftness, and have always enjoyed the sports that favored these qualities.

Now, years after graduating from high school, I still get together occasionally with Beldy Massey, who is married to Mary Ann, one of my wife's best friends. Beldy was the triple-threat athlete in my class at school — an all-state hero in basketball, football, and track. And I love to hear him tell how startled and frustrated he was, in the hundred-yard dash at a field day in our junior year, when I beat him by a couple of yards. I was still a skinny little kid, three years younger than Beldy, and he was the invincible star athlete. Yet that day I outran him.

As bodies go, mine has been a good one. I have always thrown off infections easily, and, when cut or wounded, healed quickly. Despite an unusually high cholesterol count, my heart continues to be strong and vigorous, my blood pressure is incredibly low, and my endurance is high. I have had doctors send me out to run up and down stairs before taking my pulse rate because it was so abnormally low. At the age of seventy, after experiencing a pulmonary embolism, I still managed two days later to play four sets of vigorous tennis, swim for an hour, and then enjoy a five-mile walk.

My wife laughs at the odd things that have happened in my medical history. When I was twenty-three I had a spinal fusion to repair the injury I received as the bottom man on a five-man acrobatic tower some high-school classmates and I managed to keep erect for twenty-five seconds. Spinal operations were very risky then — the survival rate was only 50 percent — and the surgeon, Dr. William K. Massie, did not like to perform them unless absolutely necessary. He particularly avoided doing them, he said, on doctors and ministers. But I was insistent, knowing that without an operation I would soon be lame from the excessive pain in my lower extremities.

Besides, I had an insurmountable faith in God that everything would be okay. And, if it wasn't, well, that was okay too, because I believed strongly in a wonderful after-life.

Dr. Massie removed the fifth lumbar-sacral disc, sawed away part of the vertebrae above and below it, and fused them together, wrapping them with a silver wire that eventually became covered by bone. The day after surgery I was up doing knee bends at the end of my bed, and, once I had shed the scar tissue on my spinal cord, never had any further trouble with my back.

At thirty-three, I had appendicitis. It made me feel terribly ill, and when I came home from class with a high fever I barely managed to crawl up the steps to the house, peel off my clothes, and tumble into bed. Anne called the doctor and he ordered her to get me to the hospital immediately. She had to badger me into getting up, and then half-carried me to the car for the trip to the emergency room. I was in surgery longer than expected because the appendix, which was on the point of bursting, had become lodged behind another organ and was difficult to remove.

At forty-five I had a rectal fistula, a strange, balloon-like bit of flesh that was gorged with blood and throbbed like a boil from hell. We were in France that year, and I went to a French proctologist who scheduled an operation the following Tuesday. On Saturday night my wife and I accompanied some friends to the Lido, and afterward to an all-night restaurant in Les Halles called *Le Chien qui fume* — The Smoking Dog. By then the fistula had become so distended that it was painful to sit on. And by Sunday morning I was out of my head with pain. Anne called Ellis Bradford, a friend who was head of City Bank in Paris and on the board at the American Hospital.

"Get him to the hospital," said Ellis, "and I'll see that the doctor is called."

The doctor happened to be at his country estate for the weekend and was greatly irritated at being summoned back early. He threw me across the bed on my stomach and lanced the fistula without benefit of anesthesia. Anne heard my scream from down the hall, where she was waiting. When she entered the room, I was chalk-white and my hands were gripping the corner of the mattress so tightly that she couldn't pry them loose. The doctor merely stuffed the wound with cotton and waited until Tuesday to complete the surgery, which thankfully was done under such heavy sedation that I didn't fully regain consciousness for twenty-four hours.

Before that episode, I spoke very fluent French. Afterward, I could barely summon enough words and phrases to get by in the marketplace, and it was a year before my fluency began to return.

When I was fifty-seven, I had a mole removed and biopsied and it turned out to be a malignant melanoma. I spent a night preparing for the worst before telling my wife what the doctor had said; I needed to be in good shape to handle her panic when she received the news. But I went to a top-flight oncologist who performed the surgery on an outpatient basis and assured me I wouldn't have any more trouble, as we had caught the problem in its early stages. The cancer was in the middle of my chest, where there isn't much flesh, but it seemed to me that he excised a great deal, and when he sewed me up I felt like a turkey that had been laced for the oven.

When I was seventy, I developed a mysterious spot on the upper lobe of my right lung that produced a persistent cough. The doctors said it didn't appear to be cancerous but ought to come out. When it had been excised, the pathologists decided it was a pulmonary embolism. I spent four days in the hospital, then threw blood clots in the affected lung and had to be treated for those. A surgeon installed a Greenfield filter, a weird, umbrella-like device made of titanium, in the vena cava to catch any more clots and put me on Heparin and Coumadin. When I left the hospital eight days later, the Heparin was discontinued. I still had a swollen leg, which the doctors said would eventually go down. But it turned out that I had a clot in that leg and had to be treated with Heparin again. This time the swelling disappeared.

Now I have a silver wire and a Greenfield filter in me, and no appendix.

But otherwise I have been an extraordinarily healthy person, and even in advancing age feel as fit and energetic as I did at forty. I continue to swim and play tennis. I go to the gym three times a week for a thorough workout, and always feel great afterward. My wife and I walk from three to six miles a day, weather permitting, and often go for a longer hike if we are in the beautiful Lake District of England. As I said, I was very fortunate to receive the genes I did.

I often look at people who have had terrible problems with their bodies, such as polio, multiple sclerosis, Parkinson's, or Lou Gehrig's disease, and marvel at their enormous courage. I wonder if I would be able to handle such diseases myself, because I enjoy my body so much. I sometimes watch Stephen Hawking or the late Christopher Reeve on television and think they should receive a thousand gold medals each for their indomitable spirits. They have borne the greatest adversity with the most remarkable aplomb, and I cannot believe that I could do as much.

Each night, during the war and aftermath of the war in Iraq, I prayed for the victims of that conflict, particularly the many soldiers on each side who were horribly burned in explosions and had to languish in hospitals as doctors and nurses tried to provide a measure of comfort and healing. And I have prayed too for the thousands of people, civilians as well as soldiers, who suffered the loss of eyes, limbs, or other parts of their bodies, and had to adjust to life on new terms. I have wondered if I could have borne their injuries as bravely and patiently as they have.

༄

Now, in my seventies, I treasure each of my body's problems across the years as something that was intimately a part of me, something that subtly but inevitably changed me and helped me to be the person I am today. Each is like a chisel mark in a piece of individually crafted furniture — part of the historical provenance on my life. I wear them like badges of honor, for they are my personal scars of existence.

I remember a story about a man who went to see Dr. Edgar Jackson, one of the founders of the modern pastoral care movement. Jackson had retired and moved to New England, and the man, who had read his books, came to him to discuss a personal problem. They talked for a while, and then Jackson led the man outside, saying he had something he would like to show him.

They walked out to a pasture surrounded by large old maple trees. Jackson explained that when those trees were young they were planted by a farmer who used them as the living posts on which he strung barbed wire to fence in his cattle. He asked the man to examine some of the trees closely. When the man did, he could see the scars where the wire had long ago become embedded in the wood.

A few of the trees, said Jackson, died from infection. But most had merely enclosed the wire and gone on growing. We have a choice, said Jackson. We can either give up because of the problems we encounter or we can elect to go on with our lives. We will always bear the scars as reminders of our encounters with the barbed wire. But they will not stop us from living life to the fullest.

I am thankful to feel that way about the things that have befallen my body. Some were life threatening, and they were all uncomfortable at the time. But none of them became the center of my existence. The scars they left remind me that they happened. But that is all. They were momentary occurrences in a life that had other things to do and other places to go.

One thing is sure. As we grow older our bodies eventually give out or begin to develop serious problems. That's merely the nature of bodies. They were not designed to last forever. As the Apostle Paul said, this mortal flesh must give way to the immortal. But until it does it is still a cooperating partner with the spirit.

᠄ᢙ

Someone once designed a birthday card with a pigeon on the front of it. Inside, there was an amorphous blob of something on the card, and the caption said, "Growing old is pigeon poop!"

There are times when I remember that and smile. Sometimes now my joints ache or I get pain down in my back from a strained muscle. I recently had cataract surgery. My brain occasionally has trouble remembering a name or a fact that I know very well is there. And I no longer feel secure climbing tall ladders, lifting heavy loads, or playing singles in tennis.

But my body is still a remarkable organism. Christopher Fry, the poet and playwright, once wrote a magnificent essay about the miracle of the hand, and how all the muscles and nerves work to make it open and shut as it does, pick up small objects, and handle an ax or a hoe. If you really want to see something breathtaking and stupendous, Fry said, just stare at your hand. Flex it a few times and consider what a marvel it is. Then think about the rest of your body — the feet, the legs, the knees, the heart, the lungs, the liver, the kidneys, the brain. What a bundle of miracles we are! And it doesn't compromise the miracle a bit that we are growing older and things don't work as flawlessly as they once did. It only proves what miracles we have been all along!

It was George Bernard Shaw who said that youth is wasted on the young. Perhaps bodies are too. I know that I appreciate my body a lot more now than I did when I was a young man. It humbles me some. But it has also become part of my spiritual appreciation of life. I thank God for it, and for all the things it has done in a lifetime. I am not sure what the Apostle Paul meant about our bodies being suddenly transformed when we die, in the blink of an eye. He may have had in mind an indescribable transmutation, a quantum leap from being physical persons to being entirely spiritual souls. I would certainly like to take my body along when I die, because it has been such a good friend all these years. I don't fancy leaving it behind like cast-off clothing, although that is apparently how it works. I am not sure if I will know how to be me without it. It is at once my grounding and my limitation, my base of resources and my restriction. Our fate has been linked for many years. It does not seem fair of me to go off without it.

Over the years, I have often thought of Samuel Beckett's little play *Krapp's Last Tape*. Krapp is an old man — I think the scatalogical name was intended — who sits on the stage listening to reels and reels of tape he has recorded through the years. He has been a philosopher, and much of the talk on the tapes now strikes him as mere drivel, so he often hits the "fast-forward" button and whirs ahead. The places on the tapes where he usually pauses to listen are from the times when he was with a woman, as in this fragment we hear about a time when he was with a girl in a punt: "...my face in her breasts and my hand on her. We lay there without moving. But under us all moved, and moved us, gently, up and down, and from side to side." Again and again Krapp returns to such memories of love and the body. They alone appeal to him now that he is older. The philosophy is all suspect, and makes him cross. But the flesh — ah, the flesh is another matter!⁴

Which brings us back again to the matter of sexuality. . . .

≈

One cannot think about the body without thinking about sex. The body *is* sex, however much some people will deny it. It was made for sex, the Apostle Paul notwithstanding. In the newborn baby lies the seed of another child, and in that one the seed of another, and so on. We cannot avoid the fact that we are like the animals and the plants of the world when it comes to that. We are here to procreate, to make certain that our species continues. Therefore we are sexual beings from the very beginning. If we do other things, such as build skyscrapers, paint portraits, compose symphonies, and manufacture plumbing materials, it is only incidental; sex has first claim on us.

Maybe our doing these other things is only an additional expression of our sexuality. Freud was right in that: how we feel about sex, whether we express it easily or repress it, whether we are comfortable with it or wish, like the man who was given one talent only, to bury it in the ground and not be troubled by it, determines almost everything about us. That sounds extreme, but it isn't. We are living, walking, breathing sex machines. Sex is our fate, and we cannot finally escape it.

In her book *Two-Part Invention,* which focuses on her relation with her husband, Hugh Franklin, Madeleine L'Engle tells about the couple's love life and devotion to one another. In the end, when Hugh was dying of cancer in a hospital, and Madeleine had to go home alone at night, she said they were "making love during this time in a profound way." He was making love with her "in the pressure of his fingers," and she with him by doing "simple little bodily services." And that, she said, was "intercourse as much as the more usual ways of expressing our sexuality."[5] It was. It was muted and subdued, to be sure. But those were nonetheless acts of sex.

There is a similarly touching passage in Browning Ware's *Diary of a Modern Pilgrim.* Ware's wife, Juanell, had Alzheimer's. He tells about her visit home for Thanksgiving a few months after she entered a residence for Alzheimer's patients. Some neighbors shared their Thanksgiving dinner with them. Juanell dropped her first bite of food and then spilled milk as she attempted to recover it.

"Later, our before-bed shower became a circus — two old people, half-stumbling, trying to get the hot water just right. Then, bed clothes. We laughed as I tried to make her adult diaper fit comfortably. Medicine next — hers and mine. Finally, love-making — gentle hand-holding for 20 or 30 seconds before. . . .

" 'I love you.'

" 'I love you, too, darling.'

"Then sleep."[6]

Young people might see nothing very sexual in all this, but older folks will understand. Our lives are crammed with sex from first to last. It differs in the various segments of our lives. But it is always there as a profound force, even in the lives of the greatest saints.

৩

I marvel now, in old age, at the irrepressibility of erections I sometimes got as a pubescent boy while merely walking down the street. My genitals would rub against the crotch of my pants and I would be embarrassed to realize that my emerging manhood was pressing like a flagpole against the front of my trousers. I changed my gait, and even my manner of walking, trying to relieve myself of the stimulation. Usually it worked. When it didn't, I had to remove my jacket and carry it in front of me.

It was as impossible in those days not to think of girls I saw — girls in their tight-fitting skirts and sweaters — as mating machines. I tried not to regard them that way, but my unconscious mind was always atwitter about it, as if some underground spring were constantly roiling up from the depths and disturbing the otherwise placid surface of my thoughts.

Our preacher wagged his finger at us and scolded us about "all the dark thoughts" in our heads, promising divine retribution if we didn't banish lustful yearnings. The text was burned into my memory, "If thine eye offend thee, pluck it out." I understood later, when I read Karl Menninger's *Man Against Himself,* about all the patients Menninger had seen who had burned or castrated themselves in last-ditch efforts to avoid damnation.

But as soon turn back a river as quench the heat of desire in a healthy young person, because nature itself designed us as sensual creatures whose most basic need is to reproduce our kind. Sex is really an itch to fulfill the commandments of nature. When the commandments of God appear to take sides against those of nature, an inevitable tension occurs, especially in the person who is religious — a tension that cannot be resolved until the conflict in ideologies itself is resolved.

It is entirely possible that my wife and I married as young as we did — I was barely nineteen and she seventeen — in order to resolve the conflict. At the time we believed it was because we came from homes where there was too much wrangling and too little love. But who knows, on reflection, whether that wasn't only a sublimation of a more basic need in both of us?

I have always been grateful that my wife was and is a beautiful woman. Part Irish and part Italian, she has the wit and intelligence of one and the passion and demonstrativeness of the other. The last of seven children, with an eight-year span between her and the next oldest, she grew up essentially alone in her home, with older parents who had not wanted an additional child and often treated her as if she were not there. Thus there was a kind of quiet, brooding quality about her that only added to her attractiveness. Several of her male classmates have confessed at class reunions that they had a crush on her but were afraid to ask for a date because she appeared so mysteriously aloof. She soon learned not to be quiet and brooding, after we married, but she has never lost her beauty. At seventy years of age, she still has the figure she had at twenty, and a smile that is even more dazzling today than it was then.

Once, when we were living in Paris, she won a contest to become a model in a Procter and Gamble television ad, and spent several days being photographed on a bateau mouche sailing up and down the River Seine between Notre Dame and the Eiffel Tower. The producer tried to get her to go to Italy with him after the shoot. She smiled and said she would be glad to go if her husband and children could go too.

For me, her beauty has never paled. I have often been grateful for this, and pondered what might have happened if I had married any of the other girls to whom I was attracted. I have seen some of them across the years, and marveled at how time has faded, thickened, and generally punished most of them. But not Annie. I find her even more alluring today than she was when I married her, and we have had a wonderful, fulfilling sexual life together.

When our oldest son was twelve, she found a copy of *Playboy* hidden under his mattress. Just before his arrival home from school, she donned a low-cut body suit with black stockings and high heels, affixed some rabbit ears to her head and a big ball of cotton to her bottom, and stepped out from behind the door to greet him as a Playboy bunny. He was shocked, and, as far as we know, didn't bother to hide any more men's magazines in his room.

I took her photograph, and we still get it out and laugh over it from time to time. But aside from a few wrinkles in her face, she still looks the same, all these years later. I am one very lucky man!

One of the discoveries we have made jointly is the one so many psychologists and anthropologists are talking about today — that life isn't just about the sex act, it's about sexuality, and sexuality is something we have all our lives. It permeates everything we do, everything about us — the way we stand, the way we walk, the way we smile, the way we speak, the way we touch one another, everything. It's part of what made the *Grumpy Old Men* films enduring favorites. There is something perennially appealing about the Ann-Margrets, Sophia Lorens, Jack Lemmons, and Walter Mathaus of the world. Age doesn't stale, nor time wither, the little things that make them attractive.

For two or three years now the older generations have enjoyed the movie *Calendar Girls*, about a group of middle-aged ladies in the British Women's Institute who decide to make a revealing calendar they can sell to raise money for a hospital memorial to one of their deceased husbands. Part of the film's appeal is the dawning realization among the women, as the project unfolds, that their days of sexual attractiveness are not over. The very realization makes them young again. And seeing them return to vibrancy has a similar effect on audiences, who suddenly realize that they too still possess the chemistry to attract the opposite sex.

Doctors universally admit now that having sex is good for our health at any age — that the stimulation of the body to orgasm releases endorphins that keep us young and make us feel better. Older people, they say, live longer and have more quality in their lives if they are still engaging in sexual acts or even if they are only dating and enjoying the company of the opposite sex.

Along those lines, something very strange happened to me at the age of seventy when I had a lung operation. I was in the hospital for twelve days and spent an additional week in a motel near the hospital before I was able to travel home. When I left the hospital I was as weak as a kitten. An eight-inch incision behind my right arm temporarily left my range of motion extremely limited, and I had to have help performing such basic functions as taking a shower and cleaning myself after a bowel movement. As for sex, it was the farthest thing from my mind — or so I thought.

Six weeks after my return home, while I was still in a recuperative mode, I experienced the urge to write a novel. The idea presented itself one day while I was in the doctor's office. It was about a young middle-aged writer who went to his female doctor because he was depressed, was attracted to her, and soon proposed that the two of them have what he called "an intentional affair" — one designed for a limited amount of time, so that they would then terminate the relationship without resentment on either side. Nothing ever works out that way in real life, of course, and it didn't in the novel, which I finally felt compelled to write.

The thing that amazed me, in the novel, was the number of liaisons I described between the writer and the doctor, and how erotic they were. It was as if the novel wrote itself — and all those steamy bedroom sessions had come straight out of my own repressed psyche. I hadn't been thinking sex. If anything, I felt as if I had become a sexless creature. But there were these lurid sexual tableaux rising like hot geysers out of my subconscious and pouring themselves onto my computer screen.

I was flabbergasted! When my wife wanted to read what I had written — because I had told her about it — I was hesitant. Frankly I was embarrassed to think that these graphically written scenes had come out of my mind, and didn't want her to think I was some kind of porn freak. When with fear and trembling I did finally place the manuscript in her hands, she thought the scenes were beautifully and tastefully done, and said she had read much worse from some of her favorite novelists. That was a relief, and helped to mitigate the shame I had felt. But I am still amazed at the smoldering sexuality my mind wanted to deal with after a period of forced abstinence and incapacity.

ᴄ·ᴐ

What it all comes down to, I think, is the incredible sexuality of our existence — even those of us who have spent our lives working in the church and thinking about theology — and how in the end that must be accounted for in any kind of spirituality we have before God.

For my part, I am happy to own before God the fact of my body and its needs and desires, and to express my thanks for human sexuality as

I have experienced it. It may have been a blessing that I grew up in a conservative church where intercourse before marriage was forbidden and lust was condemned at any time, but I am grateful that I grew beyond that narrow interpretation of sensual urges and came eventually to understand how basic sex is to life itself.

I think of all the religions in which sex is encouraged, even to the point of temple prostitution, where mating with the divine whores has been connected with the experience of transcendence and doing the will of the deity. There is more truth in that than our Judeo-Christian heritage is willing to admit. I have seen too many sick people in the course of my life as a minister — people made sick by puritanical views of sexuality — to believe that we've got it all right in Christianity.

Sam Keen, the theologian turned psychologist, did get it right in *Apology for Wonder* when he said that there is something basically pathological about either the Dionysian or the Apollonian person — one extremely loose about sex and the other unnaturally restrained. The first is too blithely ignorant of the consequences of his or her acts and of the existence of evil in the world, and the second is so excessively responsible as to frequently overlook the wonder and miracle of life.

How do I feel about the rampant sexuality in today's world? Nudity, crude language, celebrity coupling, exploitative sensuality, and all the rest?

I think three things:

First, that it is the natural rebound of a world long crippled by excessive prudery and restrictiveness. Puritanism and Victorianism both held unnatural and unreasonable attitudes toward sexual behavior. Repression inevitably leads to revolution, whether in psychological, physical, or political matters.

Second, that it is very unhealthy for young people today, who are encouraged to engage in sexual thoughts and activity before they are ready for them. In primitive times, when sex was essentially free of religious restrictions, sexual behavior became truly free only when the young were old enough to hunt and provide for themselves and their families. Now children engage in full sexual activity while still receiving allowances from their parents and their parents are still helping them with their homework. That is grossly irresponsible of our society.

Third, the pendulum will one day swing back again. It isn't a matter of stuffing the genie back into the bottle. Instead, it's a matter of shifting generational patterns and an eventual recovery of social equilibrium that will permit adults to set new guidelines for sexual behavior among the young, simply as a matter of what is good for them and society. History has always careened back and forth between extremes.

But having said all that, I have to add that I am grateful to God for the insights into our true selves that have been afforded by the sexual revolution in our time. We are not terrible sinners because we have sensual thoughts and feelings. These are perfectly natural expressions of our humanity, of who we are as creatures of the world. People who are less inhibited by society's lagging sexual consciousness — those who have affairs, who engage in striptease, who manufacture or turn to pornography — are no worse than the people who maintain a course of abstinence or repression. They are certainly no worse than priests who abuse young people sexually or parents who fondle their children. Sex is powerful. It can be used for good or evil. The point is, sex is volatile and dangerous, and isn't always easy to regulate properly, so that we don't go off on tangents or indulge it to excess.

Jesus, I am happy to say, appears to have understood this even in his day. He displayed an infinite patience for the prostitutes and other sinners of his time, and admonished the self-righteous not to judge them lest they themselves be judged by standards they wouldn't like. I am very happy with the books and articles and films today that depict Jesus as a sexual being who was probably married or had a love relationship with Mary Magdalene, who was possibly a prostitute he rescued from a life of degradation. We don't know, of course. But our willingness to think of him as a normal human being with sexual needs and desires like our own is a step toward wholeness in our religious attitudes, and I applaud it.

The body is not the evil thing medieval and puritanical theology tried to make it. It is a glorious, wonderful miracle of creation, right up there on a par with sunrises and sunsets, mountain laurel, and tomatoes on the vine. Come to think of it, it is more than on a par with these things, it is far beyond them. It is one of the consummate blessings of God, and we should treasure it and be grateful for it beyond all words. And as we grow older our gratitude ought to well up in our prayers, so that in the end our bodies commend our souls to God.

Eight

And All the Dead

I woke up the other morning thinking about Vi Farnsworth. Vi — short for Viola — lived with her husband, Wesley, in a tiny, attractive cottage a few steps from our parsonage in New England. They were considerably older than we — we were still in our early twenties — and had a daughter a few miles away who was about our age. Vi and Anne became great pals while we lived there, taking frequent day trips into Boston or up to the remnant shops at the textile mills in Lawrence.

Vi had a beautiful accent, half British, half New England, half middle American. If that adds up to more than 100 percent, it's okay, because Vi had a 150-percent voice. I loved to hear her talk. Her range of inflections was enormous, and her way of inserting laughter into her words was totally charming. She had a wonderful sense of humor, and pleasure always trailed her like an aura.

I don't know why I was thinking about Vi. Maybe I had had a dream about her. She was a member of our small congregation. Wesley wasn't. He didn't boast about being an atheist, but Vi gave us the idea that he didn't believe in much of anything. He was a bank clerk in Boston, and got up to ride the train in early, then came home late. So Vi was pretty much alone except for Anne and the church. She loved her daughter but didn't see her often. I don't think they got along very well, though I couldn't imagine why. I thought Vi was the kind of person anybody would want for a mother.

As I thought about Vi, it was almost like having a conversation with her. We hadn't seen her for several years. Once, driving from Mackinac Island via Canada and down through New England, we stopped to visit friends from our old congregation and went to see Vi in the nursing home. We had a wonderful visit, renewing old memories and chatting about life in general. She was visibly much older but still the same effervescent woman with the laughing voice we had known before. I noticed that people turned their heads to see where that fabulous voice was coming from.

It's funny how you can hold people like Vi in your memory for years and years, and then visit with them in the imagination as if they were right there in the room with you. It isn't any wonder that people in certain African tribes believe when they dream about someone that the person is right there with them. Memory is that strong and serviceable. Once people are caught in the trap of our relationships they stay there forever.

My parents are like that. I can stop whatever I'm doing, think about either of them for a minute, and Mom or Dad is suddenly with me again. I don't know if they really are — if somehow, in the world beyond this one, their spirits are hovering near enough to be on call that way, or have some kind of instant messaging that zooms them immediately to wherever their beings are invoked. It's plausible, though I don't find that it really matters one way or the other.

I remember when my mother died. That night I had a dream about her. She was going on a long cruise somewhere in the tropics. A female friend was accompanying her. I went down to the port to see them off. There were palm trees over us and a gentle breeze rustled their branches. The ship was big and sleek and beautiful, and its hull loomed above us at the dock. I looked through the crowd for my mother, and when I found her she was in a very festive mood. She looked wonderful — younger than she had appeared in years — and was eager to get on her way. She was wearing a very smart outfit — one I had never seen. We hugged and kissed, and she and the other woman climbed the gangplank. They stood among all the other passengers on the deck, waving and throwing streamers and confetti as the ship sailed out of the harbor. It was a beautiful way to say goodbye.

The night my father died, I dreamed about him too. He was standing barefoot in a meadow, with his pant legs rolled up. He looked the way I remembered him as a young man, tall and thin and handsome, with a shock of dark, unruly hair falling across his forehead. Mother was coming down the hill to meet him. She too was barefoot, and looked youthful and happy. They joined hands and started off across the meadow and back up the hill. It was a beautiful sight, especially after their years of alienation, and consoled me about the loss of both parents.

A number of times over the years I have dreamed of one or both of them, and have always awakened from the dream with a wonderful sense of well-being, as if I had actually had a nourishing visit with them. I sympathize with young Emily, in Thornton Wilder's *Our Town*, who wants to return to her home for a single day and see everybody in their natural places in her life. But somehow I feel blessed with the ability to do that, to be with my parents whenever I choose, merely by stopping and thinking about them for a while.

☙

I had an experience once with my dead grandfather, John E. Killinger. My maiden aunt was showing us slides of the family, including him, and once, when she projected his picture on the screen, he suddenly became much more than a two-dimensional image. It was as if he were actually fixing us with his powerful stare. We all felt it and were shaken by it. My aunt, a big, nonsensical woman who would have pooh-poohed the story if she had heard about it instead of experiencing it, was the most shaken of all.

"He was really here, looking at us!" she said.

But I always enjoyed my maternal grandfather, Clay Ellis, more. John Killinger was a tough, hard man who had once been a sheriff in the Old West. I never felt any love or tenderness from him. But Clay Ellis — there was a love of a man!

In all his life, he lived in only two houses, the one where he was born —
a gracious, two-storey farm home in Bracken County, Kentucky, three
miles from the little community of Germantown — and the one where he
and his wife, Ina, set up housekeeping a mile down the road. There were
no living siblings when his father died, so he inherited the old home place
and eventually moved back there.

I was born in the second house, where he and Ina lived for most of
their married life. It was during the Great Depression, and my father, who
had gone to Kentucky as a county agent, was out of work. He and my
mother had to move in with her parents and Dad ran a huckster wagon, a
sort of mobile general store, to make ends meet. I was born while he was
doing that.

The thing about Clay Ellis was his gentleness. A tall, kindly looking
man who always stood ramrod straight, even in his nineties, he was quiet,
musical, slow to anger, and almost always happy. He was so generous that
he never had very much of anything. He and Ina had three children, two
girls and a boy. The two girls went to college and became teachers. The
boy was a lovable ne'er-do-well who drank too much, gambled with funds
he didn't have, and was almost always in debt. My grandfather bailed him
out so many times that the sisters stopped counting. In the end, he lost
one farm, then the other, to take care of his son. I said he lived in only
two houses. I forgot the little place to which he finally moved, in town,
because he had to let the old home place go.

My cousins and my wife always said I inherited Clay Ellis's nature. I am
very happy for that. I cannot imagine a greater gift I might have had from
him. Placid and easy-going, he seemed to like everybody — even some of
the rascals who from time to time took advantage of his good nature. He
made excuses for everybody's failures except his own.

One of my fondest memories is of the time when I visited him late in
life, when he was having some gastric problems. I drove him into town
to visit old Doc Yelton, little Germantown's only physician for fifty years.
Doc's office was like something out of *All Creatures Great and Small*. There

were bookcases around the patients' waiting room, and on top of the cases were stuffed birds — owls, pheasants, grouse, even a wild turkey. All very hygienic, of course. Papa (which is what we called my grandfather, pronouncing it "paw-paw") confided to me on the way to town that he would like to get a shot if the nurse was there to administer it, but didn't want it if she wasn't, because Doc Yelton shook when he gave shots and sometimes stabbed people more than once. It was late in the day, and the nurse had gone home. So Papa began dancing away from the idea of a shot, and asked the doctor if he didn't have some tablets that would do just as well.

Doc Yelton said yes, and took down a large, yellowish-looking bottle from the shelf and dumped out a couple of pills into his hand. He dropped the pills into a tall glass, stepped over to the sink, and filled the glass with water. "Here," he said, thrusting the glass at my grandfather, "drink this!"

My grandfather did, and handed back the glass.

The doctor looked into the glass and saw that the tablets were still at the bottom. So he filled the glass with water again, looked around his desk, came up with what I think was an obstetrical instrument, stuck it down in the glass, stirred it around, and again ordered my grandfather to drink the contents.

My grandfather did, and once more handed back the glass.

The doctor peered into the glass and saw that the tablets were still stubbornly undissolved. Once more he filled the glass. This time he picked up a pair of bandage scissors, inserted them into the glass, and carefully hacked up the tablets. Again he handed the glass to my grandfather.

"Doc," pleaded my grandfather, "you've already got me bloated up like a cow!"

"Drink it!" was the doctor's unsympathetic response.

My grandfather did, and set the glass on the doctor's desk. "What do I owe you, Doc?" he asked, taking out the worn old purse he carried in his pocket.

"Oh, fifty cents, I reckon," said the doctor.

My grandfather fished around in his purse, took out two quarters, and handed them to the doctor with thanks.

As we were going down the sidewalk from the office, the doctor stuck his head out the door and yelled after us, "Mr. Clay, don't eat any pickles for supper!" It was the last touch on a beautiful portrait of small-town Americana.

In his eighties, my grandfather began having mini-strokes that affected his eyesight, and by the time he was ninety he was nearly blind. Sitting in a rocking chair, he listened to the radio, especially when he could get the news or hear a musical program. He never complained about his lot. He was as patient as he was gentle. When he died, the church was overflowing for his funeral. "He was the kindest, sweetest man who ever lived," said everybody who spoke to me.

I'm glad to have a man like that on my side in heaven. It seems to make my praying easier.

⌒

As we get older, our lives are filled with the ghosts of old friends and family members who have passed away. I don't think of this with sadness. On the contrary, it is wonderful and beautiful. It's as if our lives were literally crowded with the spirits of the people we've known and loved.

Maybe this is one of the things I like best about J. K. Rowling's Harry Potter novels. There isn't an impassable boundary between the living and the dead in Harry Potter's world. Old ghosts, like Nearly Headless Nick, who can tug on one ear and pull his almost-decapitated head to the side, roam the halls of Hogwarts School for Witchcraft and Wizardry as freely and visibly as the students and faculty do. Occasionally they even invite their friends among the students — Harry and Ron and Hermione — to their "death-day" parties, and sing and dance and celebrate their ghostliness.

Most Christian churches don't make much of the New Testament injunction to pray for the dead, but I often do that. Almost every time I pray, in fact. I feel a solidarity with the dead — especially with my family members and former friends — that transcends the fact of their mortality. They are still a vital part of my life. Their love, their embraces, their words help to make me who I am today. Nothing as minor as physical death can separate us.

A couple of summers ago, an old friend of ours named Ann Ellers came to Mackinac Island with a tour group, and phoned us to meet her. We sat on the front porch of the Island House Hotel and talked for hours. Ann's husband, Frank, and I had started teaching together at Georgetown College in 1957.

Ann was about the only person left among our old friends at Georgetown. Frank had died a few years earlier. He had had a stroke and had been incapacitated for months before he passed away. Ralph Curry, who had been my professor and then was my office mate when I became a teacher, had died. So had Dick and Martha Scudder — Dick was in sociology — and A. G. Thompson, who was head of the music department. And Woodridge and Eve Spears.

Woodridge was the real genius on campus, a man so highly intelligent that it essentially crippled him for ordinary living. We called him "our phys-ed authority in the English department," because he was so afraid of giving a grade lower than a B that there were always long lines of jocks waiting to sign up for his courses. When reviewing a theme with a student, Woodridge would read aloud some awful sentence the student had written, look off with a dreamy cast to his eyes, and instead of commenting on a comma fault or the inanity of the language say something like, "I wonder if you were thinking about Keats' 'Ode on Immortality' when you wrote this?" The student would half-nod and Woodridge would move on to another line, where his remarks would again be as alien to the student's understanding as the last had been.

I once asked my friend Bill Ward, who was chairman of the English department at the University of Kentucky, how he was ever able to recommend Woodridge to Georgetown. Bill smiled — he had a truly warm and wonderful smile — and said thoughtfully, "Woodridge is the kind of character that every small college needs one of." Then, after a moment's pause, he added, "But only one."

Woodridge wrote truly esoteric poetry, the kind that even the experts had to ponder for days before assessing its hidden meanings. But he was a cousin of the famous Kentucky author Jesse Stuart, whose *The Thread That Runs So True* was a national best-seller, and that gave him instant status among a lot of scribblers. Also, his wife, Eve, a tall, courtly woman with impeccable manners and a lovely voice, was his indefatigable press agent. Eve knew Woodridge's qualities as a savant, and she never failed to tout them, wherever she was. If Woodridge had been a little more marketable, she would have turned him into America's poet laureate, or at least a famous writer like Wallace Stevens or Wendell Berry.

As I mentioned earlier, I went to school with Wendell Berry. We were in some graduate classes together at the University of Kentucky. Wendell was working on his master's degree, married the daughter of the chairman of the art department, and dropped out of sight for a few years, farming and going to writing classes at Stanford University in California. When he showed up again, he had a string of credits to his name and prizes he had won for various stories and collections of poems. In those days at the university, Wendell was an aw-shucks, raw-boned young man that nobody imagined would ever amount to very much. I remember one little short story he published in *Stylus*, the university's literary magazine. It was about two young boys who stuffed a huge firecracker into the bunghole of a pet crow, lit it, and released the crow. It exploded in mid-air. I thought that was funny — the sort of thing a country boy in Kentucky would know about — but never suspected that it was the preface to Wendell's international reputation.

I have to laugh when I think about another person I knew as a student. When I was at Harvard Divinity School, I often saw Harvey Cox sitting alone in the school refectory. Harvey looked even less prepossessing then than he does today — awkward, nondescript, always with his head in a book or a magazine, never with anybody else. Imagine how stunned I was when a few years later he published *The Secular City,* one of the best-selling and most-often-quoted books of the twentieth century. I heard the gossip that it was really a compilation of ideas he had gleaned from various missionary magazines in Europe, where he had gone to work for a while, and therefore only a flash in the pan. But Harvey wasn't done, not by a country mile. Over the years, he has consistently come up with fresh, ground-breaking works on modern Christianity, Pentecostalism, the relationship of Christianity to other world religions, and religion in general. Harvard University made him a professor, and he has annually drawn enormous crowds of students to his introductory religion classes — not the sort of place where one would normally expect to find many Harvard students.

Harvey and I have corresponded a few times over the years — he wrote a nice blurb for my book *God, the Devil & Harry Potter* — and I have continued to read him with pleasure and profit. We don't know one another well, but he has been a definite influence on my life. I hardly ever write social criticisms of religion or deal with the subject of world religions without thinking about him and things he has written across the years.

સ્

The point is, as John Donne once made so plain, none of us is an island to himself, and my soul today has been shaped and enriched by all these people who have meant so much to me over the years, even though many of them are now gone. I would not begin to be who I am without them. To me, they are that "great cloud of witnesses" which the Book of Hebrews describes as cheering us on in life's fabulous race. Even if they are no longer around, they are still vitally important to me, and the soul I offer up to God at the end of my life will have their chisel marks all over it!

સ્

I could hardly list the people, now deceased, whose lives have greatly affected mine without mentioning Dr. Preston Ramsey and Miss Lillian Vaughn.

Dr. Ramsey was my pastor when I was a boy growing up in the First Baptist Church of Somerset, Kentucky. A tall, dignified man who had become rather portly in his late forties, he spoke carefully and thoughtfully on all occasions, whether he was preaching a sermon or addressing you on the street. His voice was slightly nasal, especially when he raised it, as he frequently did in the pulpit, and he had a hard time saying *-th* on the ends of words. Consequently "myth" would become *myff* and "with" was always *wiff*. A learned man with a great library of books, Dr. Ramsey (or Brother Ramsey, as many people called him) had never attended seminary. He and his slender, attractive wife, Audrey (too attractive to be a minister's wife, most of the women thought!), had married when he finished college at Union University in Tennessee, and she had soon found herself pregnant. So he had to forego seminary in order to provide for his family, the way Jude Fawley did in Thomas Hardy's *Jude the Obscure,* although, unlike Jude, he never appeared to be bitter about it.

Dr. Ramsey arrived in Somerset shortly before I made the decision to enter the ministry, and after I made the decision he and I had many talks together. His own son, to his disappointment, never showed any interest in being a minister, so I think he regarded me as his proxy son in the ministry. I often went to his home for a visit, and always found him warm and receptive, although later I would realize that I had taken advantage of his and his wife's good nature by invading their space when they probably needed to be alone. The friendship of that strong, good man was extremely important to me at that delicate time of my development, and I have never forgotten what I owe to him.

The other person I mentioned, Miss Lillian Vaughn, came to First Baptist Church as the church's secretary at about the same time that Dr. Ramsey arrived. A straight, thin woman who always seemed to walk in a scurry, didn't wear makeup, and wore her graying hair short or pulled back in a bun, Lillian Vaughn was a Protestant nun if there ever was one. If any man ever showed an interest in her, she laughed a nervous little laugh intended to shame him for paying attention to her and let him know that she was married to Christ and her work.

And she was. Her job was all-consuming. Not only was she the minister's secretary and the church's general secretary, taking care of all correspondence that went out of the building, she attended all the meetings of the church (except those of the deacons and trustees, which women were not permitted to attend), taught a Sunday school class, and was in charge of the Sunday evening program called Training Union, which was designed to turn the church's young people into the leaders of tomorrow. In addition, her office was always open and she was besieged by a constant stream of visitors.

Nobody could be more sympathetic than Miss Vaughn. She wrote the textbook on sympathy. Not false sympathy, but real, honest, heartwringing concern. She *agonized* over other people's hurts and troubles. She prayed for just about everybody in the community, and especially for those who were enduring any kind of loss or difficulty. She was indeed a nun, and she kept the candles burning at all hours of the day and night.

If Dr. Ramsey was my father in the ministry, Miss Vaughn was my mother. She kept up with everything I did — *almost* everything — and praised me constantly for it. "Oh, Johnny!" she would say in her most appreciative voice, and I would always leave her office six inches taller than when I came in. Years later, I dedicated my book *Bread for the Wilderness, Wine for the Journey* to her, saying that she, more than anybody I knew, taught me how to pray. Her total selflessness and devotion to God made me think there wasn't anything the deity could really deny her.

These two wonderful saints, Dr. Ramsey and Miss Vaughn, stand tall in my personal Hall of Fame. If they aren't praying for me today, and still helping to shape my life, then I am greatly mistaken. Nobody could have had two finer influences on his or her life as a teenager.

In fact, there were dozens of older people at the First Baptist Church of Somerset who had a tremendous effect on me — the W. H. Ramsey, Srs., their son Bill and his wife, Eula, the Mavities, the Pings, Mrs. Tandy, the Barnetts, the Simpsons, the Jaspers, the Dodsons, the Curtises, Hassell and Barbara Dubose. The list could go on and on. I was very fortunate to have all those wonderful saints in my corner when I was young.

And now I am a very fortunate older man.

࿚

I cannot think of friends who are dead without mentioning David and Molly Eddie, our close British friends. We met David the first summer we spent in England, when we were staying at the Harley House Hotel in London, a remarkable bed-and-breakfast establishment a few doors from the Russell Square tube stop. David, a tall, dignified-looking Scotsman with keen, dark eyes, glasses, a moderate paunch, and no hair on the top of his head, was an assistant secretary in the British Department of Defense. His home was in Harrogate, but he spent a lot of time in London, and we happened to be at the Harley House on one of his longer visits.

David always missed his wife, Molly, and their children, Jill and Alan, when he was away, and I think our family became a surrogate for them. Our two sons were only six and three at the time, and David often sat with them in the evenings so Anne and I could go to the theater. They loved David, because he had a dramatic way of speaking, was extremely clever, and was always lots of fun.

Molly was a truly beautiful woman — a nice figure, lovely, curly hair, a pretty face with a dazzling smile, and a graceful, lilting voice that usually had the laughter of silver bells in it. She and David met in North Africa during World War II. The man Molly really loved had been killed in the war, and she married David on the rebound. They made an attractive couple, despite the fact that Molly always lamented that she couldn't feel as passionate about David as she had about her first beau.

Before we met Molly, the government had shifted David's office to Worcester, and they bought a lovely little home at Upton-on-Severn, a few miles south of Worcester. Over the years, we were often in their home, and once they traveled to the United States and spent three weeks with us in Nashville. They were wonderful, comfortable people, and our times together were always lively, filled with interesting conversation and speculation, because Molly was invariably interested in religious ideas and practices of any kind, even those of a spiritualist nature. She attended her little Anglican church in the village of Ripple, and once, when we were visiting, twisted the vicar's arm to have me do the sermon for them.

I have to laugh when I remember that occasion. At the conclusion of the sermon, I said, "Let us pray." But as all heads went down and some people slipped onto their kneeling benches, the little vicar rushed into the pulpit, announced a hymn number, and started leading the singing. I knew that there were Christian communions where the people did not pray with strangers, and assumed that I had stumbled upon one of them. But as the vicar and I stood at the door afterward, his wife apologized to me and explained that her husband was nearly deaf. When he saw me bow my head he assumed the sermon was over and rushed in to complete the service, never realizing that I had invited people to pray.

The reader that morning, I recall, was Brigadier General Peter Young, a retired military officer who had written one of the most definitive histories of World War II. He was a very dignified looking man who was almost the spitting image of Colonel Harlan Sanders, the founder of the Kentucky Fried Chicken restaurants, little white goatee and all, and he had a very commanding voice which he used to superb effect in reading the scriptures. I felt almost like a country hick when I mounted the pulpit after the Gospel reading to preach the sermon.

Following the service, we all retired to the vicarage for a glass of sherry before going to lunch. It was very civilized, and the vicarage, only two or three years old, was magnificent. The vicar and his wife, unfortunately, did not live there long before it was time for him to retire. When he did retire, I heard afterward, they had no money set aside, so had to go and live with a son and his wife, as his pension paid only twenty-five hundred pounds a year.

Molly and David, to our continuing sadness, both died of cancer, probably because they were heavy smokers during the war. Molly went first, with cancer of the pelvis, and David died three or four years later from cancer of the throat. Lamentably, both could have been saved if they had received proper medical treatment from the onset of their problems, but they were far too passive, we believe, in accepting the decisions — and the scheduling — of Britain's nationalized health-care system. Going to England hasn't ever been the same for us since they died.

⌡⌠

Of all the professors I had across the years — there must have been at least a hundred! — there were two who had an influence on my life surpassing all the others, and both are now dead.

One was Ralph Curry, whom I mentioned before as an English teacher at Georgetown College. I spent my second year of college at Georgetown, and Ralph was my teacher for the survey course in English literature. He was young at the time, barely out of graduate school at Penn, and thin as a rail, which he would remain for the rest of his life. Ralph's father had been a longtime, much-revered professor at Campbellsville College in Kentucky, and his brother Leonard became a history professor, so the teaching genes must have been strong in their family.

Ralph had a headful of thick, dark hair and wore rimless glasses. He was so skinny that he actually looked fragile. He wore bow ties and suits or sport coats and trousers — usually the latter. And his shoes, always brown whatever the color of his outfit, were invariably in need of polishing. His voice was strong. It was also different. I don't know quite how to characterize it. It sounded a little nasal but not unpleasantly so. He spoke rapidly and his words were carefully, precisely enunciated. He *sounded* very bright and intelligent, which he was.

I love English literature, and would probably have liked it in spite of the teacher — but Ralph had a way of making it all come alive. Not by fastidious attention to the details of biography or the rules of writing, but by humorous little asides or a subtle, clever underlining of the ideas that struck him as deep and important. Time always flew by in his classes, for he was an entertainer as well as a teacher. He knew how to make the material come alive, how to give it an occasional boost where it needed it and make it sparkle for his students.

When I graduated from Baylor University the following year, I was only nineteen and didn't feel mature enough to go directly to seminary. If I could spend a year studying English literature, I thought, I might one day become as urbane and knowledgeable as Professor Curry. That was when I decided to apply to the University of Kentucky, take a rural pastorate, and spend at least a year getting a master's degree in English. As it turned out, I enjoyed the graduate program so much that I stayed on for a doctorate. And to the extent that getting that advanced degree in English changed my life — which it did almost beyond estimate — I have always credited Ralph with the decision to do it.

When I graduated from Harvard with a degree in ministerial studies and couldn't find a Baptist pastorate that wanted me, I decided to go back to Georgetown and teach for a while. I was delighted when the dean of the college, looking for a place to stick me in an office, assigned me to one with Ralph. Seven years had elapsed since I had had him as a professor, but nothing had changed except that now I was a teacher and he was a little older. Being a little older, he was also less inhibited by the sacred halls of learning, and had become even wittier and more irrepressible than I remembered. I wish now that I had made a notebook of all the clever things I heard him say while I was his office mate.

I do, however, remember one comment in particular. Ralph was a very untidy person. Not about himself. Personally he was always neat and clean. But his office space was an unmitigated disaster. His desk was so piled with books and papers that he could rarely find anything without a prolonged search. Whenever I teased him about this, he invariably responded with a quote from Ralph Waldo Emerson, that "a foolish consistency is the hobgoblin of little minds."

ᚼ

The second professor who had enormous influence in shaping my life was George A. Buttrick, my homiletics and church-administration professor at Harvard. (His official title was Preacher to the University and Plummer Professor of Christian Morals, and he always claimed that he had once been introduced as the Moral Professor of Christian Plumbing.) Buttrick had an illustrious career before retiring to Harvard. Originally a Congregationalist from England, he had come to this country and mutated into a Presbyterian, eventually receiving an appointment as senior minister of the wealthy Madison Avenue Presbyterian Church in New York. Constantly invited to lecture at prestigious gatherings around the world, he published numerous scholarly books and edited the important multi-volume *Interpreter's Bible,* which has since been an indispensable aid to thousands of ministers. He also found time to serve as moderator of the General Assembly for the United Presbyterian Church.

But I had never heard of George Buttrick. It was an era of great professors at Harvard Divinity School. The biggest name of all was Paul Tillich, the existentialist theologian who was in the process of writing his brilliant multi-volume *Systematic Theology* and was, with Karl Barth, Rudolf Bultmann, and Reinhold Niebuhr, one of the four most important theologians in the world. Tillich's presence was the primary reason I chose to go to Harvard. But Amos Wilder and Krister Stendahl were there in New Testament, and Frank Cross Jr. and George Ernest Wright, both experts in the recently discovered Dead Sea scrolls, had currently come in the field of Old Testament. James Luther Adams and Paul Lehmann were teaching ethics, and George Huntston Williams and Heiko Obermann were the world-famous church historians. *Buttrick, smuttrick,* I thought. I had never run into his name. He couldn't possibly be very good!

Even my first class with Buttrick didn't change my mind. He was such a funny, eccentric little bird! His mannerisms were a stitch. He ducked his head as he read from his lecture notes, and made humorous little remarks that you knew weren't ad-libbed but were actually jotted in the margins, because they always had a kind of rehearsed quality about them. Then he threw his head back and walked away from the lectern as he shrugged his shoulders, like a man on short stilts, and continued talking in a rapid-fire way, delivering precise little dicta about preaching or worship or whatever it was he was discussing.

"This guy wouldn't ever make it in a Southern Baptist church," I remember saying to myself. "He doesn't have the looks or the voice or the poise to cut it in a really competitive situation."

Only gradually, over one semester and then another, did I begin to realize who this man was — and not only who he was, biographically, but who he was in stature and ability. All the things he talked about began coalescing in my mind. I knew that he knew about a lot of things I had never even encountered but was probably going to encounter in my ministry, and I began to take notes like mad. He was proud of himself, to be sure — was always tossing off casual references to people he knew. Like Emily Post, the manners guru. He rode up in an elevator with her once, and had the temerity to correct a minor faux pas in her behavior. He rattled off the names of important people in New York who had served as ushers and deacons at Madison Avenue Presbyterian Church, and observed: "It changes a man's personality when you stick a carnation in his buttonhole and send him down the center aisle of a church."

Buttrick was rarely self-deprecating. Langdon Gilkey, the eminent Chicago theologian, once served as a student intern at Madison Avenue Presbyterian Church while Buttrick was the minister there. He remarked that George Buttrick got up every morning, looked in the mirror, wrestled with his ego — and lost!

I remember the delight Buttrick took in telling about the time he wrote an Easter article for one of the big New York magazines — either *Life* or *Look,* I can't remember which — and a hard-boiled editor who called himself an atheist was proofing his material. According to another editor sitting nearby, Buttrick reported, the hard-boiled one was seen to wipe away some tears as he commented, "Say, this is damned good!"

But if Buttrick was truly proud of himself, he had strong reasons. His sermons — tight, poetic, well-argued, extremely forceful — were among the best I ever read or heard. At Harvard he commanded overflow crowds, something probably unprecedented for a university chapel in modern times. Students flocked to his office. He had a famous opening gambit with those who stumbled in and blurted out that they didn't really believe in God. "Tell me," he would say, offering the student a cigar, "about this God you don't believe in. Maybe I don't believe in him either."

After Harvard, Georgetown, and Princeton, when I had become dean of Kentucky Southern College in Louisville, I invited Buttrick to give the first annual lectures at the college. He was as much of a smash there as he had been at Harvard. People pinched themselves to be sure they really were hearing the wonderful things coming from the lecturer. I told him during his visit that I didn't intend to remain in college administration much longer. That very day, he telephoned Dean William Finch at Vanderbilt Divinity School and said he had a former student he'd like to see in the preaching post at Vanderbilt. Dean Finch called me, Anne and I drove to Nashville, and our lives changed forever.

What did I learn from George Buttrick? I learned the craft of sermon-making — that it isn't enough to have something to say and get up and say it, but it's essential to ponder it and think about ways of expressing it and then work at the manuscript until it is said as cogently and memorably as possible. I learned that the writing of prayers is as important as the writing of sermons. In fact, Buttrick always said that if he had time to write only one or the other, he would write his prayers and not the sermon. I learned that church administration is pretty much like administration anywhere else — that church workers can be as selfish and obstinate and ego-centered as corporate employees or factory hands, and that the person who runs the organization has to know what he or she is doing and do it without letting sentiment interfere with efficiency. I learned that the minister's life is far more effective if it is a life of strict self-discipline, and you read-read-read and think-think-think all the time about the tasks at hand.

Tillich and Stendahl and Frank Cross and all those other people at Harvard were important in my life — but none half so important as this cocky little Britisher who in my case overcame the handicap that at first I hadn't even heard of him!

How did Harvard affect me spiritually? At the time, I didn't really think that it did. But over the years I saw that it had made a great difference in my life. These people taught me to really *think* about faith, and that thinking about it both refines and transforms one's faith. A lot of seminaries are better worshiping communities than Harvard Divinity School was, and provide a lot more camaraderie for their students. But these men (there weren't any women at that time) gave me the tools for examining my faith, for getting a proper perspective on it, and this subtly but surely changed the way I have faith. Eventually I became very bold in my expression of faith — I had confidence in how I was analyzing and talking about it — and was able to define it with precision and individuality. If I were asked to say what Harvard did for me, it gave me courage, the same kind of courage I think being with Jesus gave his disciples.

༺༻

Today we had sad news about two dear friends.

Harold Raasch was one of the good guys in our church in California. A former restaurateur, he has worked for the last few years — since retirement — at Forest Lawn, the big L.A. cemetery. Tall, a little overweight, with closely cropped hair and a permanently red face from high blood pressure, Harold looked a lot like Jessica Fletcher's doctor-friend Seth in *Murder, She Wrote*. He was always vivacious, fun loving, compassionate, and honest. He and his wife, Harriet, were as kind and supportive as two people could possibly be.

The night before we moved from L.A., Harold showed up at our door with our dinner and a little heart-shaped necklace for Anne. He handed them to us, then stood in the doorway and cried, unable to speak. We've never forgotten that. For a guy who worked in a hard profession, he was so *human,* so *caring.* He reminded us that God mediates himself to us through our friends and loved ones.

Harold has pancreatic cancer and it is in its final stages. He will die before this book comes out.

The other friend was Jim McClenney, who died this morning. Jim was a member of the little church I served in New Jersey while teaching and doing graduate work at Princeton. A former pro-baseball player, Jim was a giant of a man. I never asked, but I'm sure he stood about six-six, with a frame to match the height.

When we met Jim and his wife, Lou, Jim was already an executive in the shipping department of Coca-Cola and Minute Maid. A few years after we were together in New Jersey, he was promoted to vice president in charge of shipping and moved to Orlando, Florida.

Lou once called me and broke into tears on the phone. She needed to see me, she said. Something was deeply troubling her. I drove to their house immediately, which was about fifteen miles from Princeton. Lou, a pretty, baby-faced, redheaded woman, had obviously been crying for hours. I couldn't imagine what her problem was. It obviously concerned Jim. Had she been unfaithful to him and was she afraid to tell him? Had he been unfaithful to her?

"I have never really loved Jim," she burbled. "It is wrong for me to go on living with him."

Pardon me? They had two children, young Mike, who was about twelve, and Lori, an adopted girl of three or four. Jim worshiped Lou. What in the world was she talking about?

Lou had been in a TB hospital for several years. She had had one lung removed, and was always a little sickly. Jim had met her there, fallen in love with her, and proposed. She married him, thinking she would come to love him. He was such a big old puppy dog, it shouldn't be hard. But she didn't feel that she had ever managed really to fall in love with him, and now it was tormenting her.

I assured her that it wasn't wrong to stay married to Jim. He needed her, I said. She gave a purpose to his life. And there wasn't anybody who would ever be as good to her as Jim.

Lou accepted that judgment, and they stayed together. When we built a new home in Nashville, Tennessee, they came with another couple, Dean and Keitha McAdoo, and spent Thanksgiving with us to christen the house. Later we visited them in Orlando.

Then Lou died. Jim was distraught. None of us thought he would ever be happy again.

But a few years later he met Barbara. Barbara was a wedding coordinator. Very chic. Dark-headed, trim, elegantly turned out — very different from Lou. Someone who knew both Barbara and Jim kept telling Jim he ought to have at least one date with her to see if he liked her. He kept demurring. But finally he capitulated and called her.

The evening of their date, he approached the front door and stood there, debating whether to ring the bell or to leave. Finally he pushed the button. The bell sounded inside and Barbara came to the door. Jim turned abruptly on his heels and walked back toward the street.

"My God," thought Barbara, "he didn't like me already!"

Halfway out the sidewalk, Jim stopped, slapped his thigh, and exclaimed "Hot damn!" Then he turned and came back to the house. They were married a few months later. It was characteristic of Jim. He was a great fellow, with a formidable sense of humor.

Three or four years ago Jim and Barbara attended a wedding for Dean and Keitha McAdoo's son at Grand Canyon. I was going to do the service, with a beautiful bride and groom who looked as if they'd stepped out of the pages of *Bride* magazine just to be photographed against the gorgeous colors of the canyon. The night before, there was a trail ride with a barbecue at the end of it. Barbara was enchanted — she loved horses. Jim didn't think he'd be comfortable on a long ride, so he opted to make the trip on the hay wagon. My Anne did too, and they sat beside one another on a bale of hay.

While we were on the trail, the individual riders on one route and the wagon passengers on another, a gully-washing thunderstorm came up. Those of us on horseback had ponchos in our saddle rolls. Those on the wagon had none. When we arrived at the barbecue site the rain had ended, but the people on the wagon were drenched. Anne said Jim groused about it all the way to the barbecue and his remarks kept everybody in stitches. His humor was always understated and infectious.

Now Jim has gone to the great roundup. We won't be sad for very long. He had a lot of things wrong with him. I'm sure he loved Barbara, and Barbara loved him. She will miss the old guy. But Anne's first remark, after she told me the news, was that now he'll be with Lou. I don't know about such things, but I'd like to think she's right. Maybe Lou was waiting for him.

Jim and Harold. They're nearly the same age — Jim in his middle seventies, Harold in his eighties. Both big men. Both extremely amiable and friendly. Both generous and humorous. Both men we hate to lose.

And yet we haven't really lost them. Their spirits are still part of our entourage, part of our *nepheshes*, and always will be.

෴

I knew both of these men through having been their minister. That makes me realize how many of the people who still mean a lot to me have been given to me in that way — dear souls whose lives were intertwined with mine because I happened to be the minister of their churches.

Like Pauline Gover, the jolly, overweight lady in my very first parish, at Bronston, Kentucky. Mrs. Gover — she was in her fifties and I was only eighteen — was a nurse at the Somerset City Hospital, and commuted every day from the little farm where she and her husband had lived together until his death. Her son John and his wife, Ruth, lived on an adjacent farm and John looked after both properties. Another son, David, was only twelve and lived at home with her. And John and Ruth had a son named James Arthur, who was about ten, and a three-year-old named Anthony. We ate with the Gover family, at Pauline's or John and Ruth's, more than with any other family in the congregation, and there was always a lot of love and laughter around the table, as well as an abundance of good food.

One night we were having supper at John and Ruth's house when all the shades were pulled. The reason they were drawn is that a prisoner had just shot a policeman only a few miles away and was believed to be on the loose in our vicinity. He was armed and obviously dangerous, and everybody was on pins and needles until he was recaptured. Halfway through the meal there was a sharp rap at the front door. We all bolted like a bunch of rabbits. The women stayed in the kitchen with Anthony. I found a ball bat, and, with John, James, and David, proceeded cautiously to the door. When we opened it, a young boy stood there.

"Can James Arthur come out and play?" he asked in a squeaky little voice.

We returned to the kitchen to find my wife, Anne, sandwiched so tightly between the refrigerator and a counter that she couldn't get out until we helped her. We all collapsed in laughter over her predicament. It was typical of the good times we had together.

There are so many people I remember fondly, as I do the Govers. At Poplar Grove Baptist Church, my other rural parish in Kentucky, there were Ed Cook and his wife, Myrtle, the only college graduates in the congregation. Myrtle's dear little mother, Mrs. Farley, who was bright as a new penny and had dozens of people in for Sunday dinner after she was well into her nineties. Willie and Docie Creech. Willie had been a coal miner in West Virginia, and carried a pistol to work during the tumultuous days when John L. Lewis was trying to organize miners into a union to fight for better pay and working conditions. Ian Kirby (everybody pronounced it *een*) and his quiet, beautiful little family, who lived next to the church. Ian always built the fire in the church's woodstove during the winter months, and once or twice, when the roads were nearly impassable with snow or ice, he and I were the only ones in attendance.

Myrtle Cook was an inordinately heavy woman who looked almost exactly like Hyacinth Bucket's sister Daisy on *Keeping Up Appearances,* only twice as fat. She had a disconcerting habit of belching loudly in the middle of a prayer in the Sunday service. Eventually the doctors discovered that she had a leak in her small intestine and operated to repair it. We thought that would stop her untimely eruptions, but apparently the habit was too ingrained to break.

Willie Creech was a delightful man who still spoke with some of the archaisms he had grown up with in West Virginia. He thanked God for having "hoped" us, and for all the blessings he had "stowed-ed down" upon us. And he was as Godfearing and generous and funny as any man I've ever known. Once, when he and his wife had boarded a visiting preacher for a week, he asked me casually at dinner after that, "Preacher, do you remember that fellow Buddy who stayed with us while he was preachin' at the church?"

I said I did.

"Well," said Willie, "every afternoon when I went down to get the cows, I found him standing there a-preachin' to them — practicin' his sermon, I reckon."

There was a pause.

Then he added, "You know, preacher, them cows ain't milked right since!"

⁓

I was reading the Sunday edition of the *Washington Post* this afternoon, and paused over the obituary pages. I'm not sure why, but lately I've made a habit of looking at the obituaries. Not because I'm getting older and wonder how my picture might look in there some day. But maybe because I feel a kindness and sympathy for the people who have lost their loved ones and post their photographs and something about them in the paper. I always pray for the families of the people I see there.

This afternoon I was attracted to the picture of a pretty girl named Amy Elisabeth Edgerton, who died back in 1987 at the age of seventeen. (A lot of people use the obituary page to remember loved ones for years after their deaths.) Amy could have been a movie star, she was so lovely. Beautiful smile, and smiling eyes as well. Nicely coiffed hair, with pretty bangs on her forehead. I'm sure her family was grief stricken when she died. Still are, apparently.

I liked the little poem they placed under her picture, name, and dates. I had never seen it before, and have no idea whether somebody in the family wrote it or it came from another source. It talked about looking at the stars and realizing that a lot of them actually died a long time ago, even though we still enjoy seeing them. The same is true of a loved one, it said, because "starlight, like love, never dies."

That's the secret, isn't it? Love never dies. The people we've cared about, the ones who have meant most to us, don't entirely desert us when they die. They seem to, for a while, because we can no longer see them or touch them when we want to. But then their memories come back to us, warm and loving and intimate, and we realize they aren't entirely gone at all. They're like the starlight that keeps shining on us year after year.

Somehow, we all live in the great love and providence of God — even those who have preceded us in death. As Alfred North Whitehead once said, "God is a tender care that nothing be lost." Nothing at all! We — the living and the dead — are bound together in love. A love that will never be broken.

I believe this with all my heart.

Nine

A World of Mystery and (Divine) Intrigue

From the earliest time I can remember, the world was to me a place of wonderful and almost unbearable mystery. I have always wondered if this was due in part to the fact that I was nearsighted and saw the world only fuzzily until I got my first pair of glasses. Whatever the reason, I now treasure it, because it is an awesome way to view everything. Even after I acquired glasses, I liked taking them off, particularly at Christmas, and seeing all the lights as warm, exploding haloes instead of in their less spectacular precision. And I have always enjoyed viewing the world in the same way, disdaining science and precision for mystery and beauty.

When I was small and played under my favorite spirea bush at the side of our house, or crawled through the tall, moist crimson clover in the garden, it was as if the entire universe around me were lush and full and secretive. Plants throbbed with a juicy life of their own and tiny insects crawled over them in an empire unknown to human beings. Each Sunday in the comic strips there was a half-page picture of life as seen by a community of little people, like Gulliver's Lilliputians, crawling about over some enormous implement discarded in the full-sized world, such as a teapot or an old soup ladle, and getting ropes over it to haul it away and utilize it for their own purposes. I loved entering their world in my imagination and viewing everything from their perspective. When I was about six my fondest wish was for a tiny airplane with an open cockpit that I could use to swoop and dive around our neighborhood, looking down on the houses and treetops, and landing safely under the old walnut tree in our side yard.

Once, after I had had the measles and been quarantined for three whole weeks, I emerged onto our front porch wearing sunglasses — my mother insisted on this precaution — to find that winter had departed and spring had arrived, with jonquils, violets, forsythia, spirea, and apple trees blooming all over the neighborhood. My little heart swelled with the fullness of the spring air itself, and garnered scents and colors with a greediness I don't think I had known before. Had the sky ever been so blue or the grass so green? Had the forsythia bushes ever flared in such brilliant yellow? It was as if the sun had poured itself into their branches and they were still sticky and alight with its pollen. I sat for the longest time in the swing on the porch — I was told not to go out into the yard — feeling more reverence for the universe than any priest ever felt in the Holy of Holies!

And when I first got glasses, it was as if the intensity of everything had been turned up a hundredfold! Wearing the new glasses, I could actually see for the first time the leaves on the trees and the stones in the walls I passed. I could see them before, of course, but only when I was practically rubbing my nose against them. Now I could make them out quite clearly at a distance, and felt overwhelmed by their intricacy. Imagine all those young green leaves sprouting at once on a single tree, and the beauty of that wall, where the workmen had forced the mortar to extrude a little from the surface of the stones like a network of hardened lace! And the clouds in the sky, which I had seen only hazily, as in a painting by Monet, were now sharply articulated.

☙

My expanding sense of the world and its mysteries was gratified when we moved shortly after that to Somerset, Kentucky, where my father had received an appointment as head of the U.S. Employment Service. As it was during World War II, no homes were being built and there was almost no housing available. Consequently we rented a collapsing old mansion on Columbia Street that sat in the middle of a vast, overgrown yard littered with fallen limbs, bottles, tin cans, newspapers, and other detritus. My father was handy with tools and soon had the house in reasonable shape. And together we cleared off the yard, hauling away load after load of debris until everything looked neat and livable again.

I loved that old house where, for the first time in my life, I had my own room, a large, mostly bare space with a bed, a lamp stand, and an abundance of windows. From the windows I could crawl out onto the tin roof over the back porch, which gave me an incredible sense of freedom and openness. And I especially enjoyed a gigantic holly tree in the front yard whose branches grew thickly at intervals of only a foot or two and thus afforded a virtual ladder from the ground to the top, some fifty or sixty feet above. I had graduated from my old spirea bush to this magnificent tree, and frequently climbed all the way to the final branches, where I would sit for hours, imagining myself invisible and feeling as if I were at the very peak of the world!

A Freudian, I am sure, would have great fun with my penchant for imaginary airplanes and this perching near the tip of an arboreal erection. Maybe it was all related to subconscious sexual awakening, I don't know. What I do know is that I was in my element at times like this, for I seemed to be then most in harmony with nature and the world around me, and felt joyously content with whatever inchoate emotions were flooding through my youthful consciousness. At that time, I didn't understand the meaning of holiness — it was a concept quite alien to my young mind — but what I felt, I have since realized, was a presence as holy as any I have ever known.

My world was crushed when I came home for lunch one day to learn that we were being evicted. The owner of the grand old house, the enormous yard, and the giant holly tree had sold the property without even offering my father a chance to bid on it, and we had only a few months in which to find another home. I couldn't eat a bite of food after hearing the news. I gloomily dragged myself back to school. I hated the owner of the house, whom I personally had never seen, for producing such unbearable anguish in my heart.

The mourning continued for weeks. I climbed the old holly tree in search of solace, and talked to it as if it were a human being, saying how much I would miss it and how wrong it was of the house's owner to dispossess us as he was doing. I think I even promised to sneak back to the tree at night, wherever we had gone, and climb it again, like a lover returning to his beloved.

Then one day my father took us for a Sunday afternoon ride in the country, and pulled off the road onto a graveled parking space near a small brick house. "Let's get out," he said. "There's somebody here I have to see."

We walked up the path to the house and stood on the porch, waiting for someone to answer my father's knock.

A small, shriveled man appeared inside the screen door, peered out, and opened it. "Come in," he said in a funny nasal voice, as if expecting us.

My father made no announcement. It dawned on me only as he and this man conversed — the man's name was Walter Leigh — that he was buying the house. I saw him pull out his wallet and hand Mr. Leigh a dollar as a sign of their agreement. They discussed a date of occupancy. My father asked how Mr. Leigh's new house was coming. "Oh, it's coming along right well," said the little man. "I've got most of the brick work done. Should get to the trim in a few days."

I can't remember if my father explained it later or I merely absorbed the fact in some more indirect way, but Mr. Leigh was a bricklayer and had built a number of houses in the area, including the one he was selling to my father. He had a small piece of property a few miles up the road and was completing another home there. He was a no-frills bricklayer, not a fancy one like the men who erected grand homes in town. And he was multitalented, so that he could build the framing, do the plumbing and wiring, and trim out the house himself. What he built didn't look fancy, but it was sturdy and, more important in a time of scarce housing, entirely livable.

Almost instantly, in the magic of this new place — which to my delight
I learned had seven acres of ground, including a spring, a pond, a barn, and
a chicken house — I forgot my grief at leaving the big old house in town
and my beloved holly tree. Here there were hills to climb, hundreds of
big, tall trees to admire, a barn whose loft was as entrancing as any place
I had ever visited, a pond filled with living creatures — tadpoles, frogs,
fish, and turtles, plus occasional ducks and geese — and, just beyond the
lower fence, a small creek that swelled into a raging torrent after a rain.
To my mystical young heart, it was more than Shangri-la, it was a veritable
outpost of heaven itself!

I could not wait until we moved. One day I hiked out to our new home,
a distance of about three miles, knocked timidly at the door, and asked
Mr. Leigh if it was all right for me to go down to the spring and the pond.
"Oh, sure," he said in his good-natured way. "It's yours now, or soon will
be. Make yourself at home. Come any time you want to."

So I became a frequent visitor, especially on weekends. I never went
to the house again, not wanting to disturb the Leighs, but always went
directly to the barn and the springhouse and the pond beyond them. There
were cows in the pasture around the pond, and I was wary of them, because
I wasn't ever quite sure if they welcomed my intrusion. But I hiked over
the hills, following little trails they had made in their wanderings, and
sat on outcroppings of rock above the pond. Once, intent on following
the cows' path through some high weeds, I passed under a cedar tree and
suddenly found myself staring eyeball-to-eyeball with three long, green
snakes hanging from the lowest branch. My heart stopped for a moment,
but apparently they were as scared as I was, for they quickly withdrew
into the foliage. I ducked to pass and didn't come that way again, not
wishing to repeat the experience on an occasion when they might not be
so obliging.

I could hardly wait until we moved!

&

Those years on that little Kentucky farm were amazingly formative for my entire life. I have told how I lost my little sister there one rainy Saturday morning when a truck hit her, killing her instantly. It is a wonder that my parents didn't sell the place after that and move away. But they didn't. Perhaps they wanted to remain near the site where Jo had died. I am glad we did stay, for the joy I drew from that wonderful little acreage has continued to nourish me to this day.

People who haven't lived with farm animals during their early years don't know what they missed. At various times we had ducks, chickens, geese, cows, pigs, and goats, but the goats were my favorites. When we first moved to the country my Iowa relatives sent me a check for twenty-five dollars to buy a pig. I think they wanted me to become a farmer, and thought this would start me in that direction. But my father decided to acquire goats before pigs, as they would be useful to keep the land clean of weeds and brush, so I invested in one of the female Toggenburgs he bought, with the understanding that I would have my pick of her first litter. She had two kids the first time she was bred, and I chose the comelier of the two, a little beige beauty with a white star on her forehead.

"What'll you call her?" my Dad asked.

"Cindy," I said, thinking of Cinderella, because I knew she would grow up to be a lovely goat.

Cindy was one of the finest pets I ever had. Finicky to a fault — goats are actually very clean animals, and ours wouldn't eat from a pan that hadn't been washed — she behaved like the young princess I thought she was. When I sat on the rocks near the barn, she would leap up beside me and, cuddling against my body, nudge me under the chin until I stroked her back.

Dad was right about the goats keeping the farm clean. Within a few weeks they had the whole place looking as if someone had gone over it with a lawnmower, and had devoured all the smaller bushes and shrubs on the hillside, mostly sassafras plants from which we sometimes dug up the roots to make medicinal tea. Then they went to work on the bark of the cedar trees that grew copiously where bird droppings had planted their seeds. And when that delicacy was about gone, one of the goats, a smart Nubian that we called Nancy after my dad's mother, not my sister, would stand on the hillside above a tree, put her front hooves against it, and bend it down so that the others could chew off the needles. Soon there weren't any more small cedars on the place.

Eventually we sold the goats because they were too much for my parents to care for with their growing business. I was sad to see them go, but also relieved, as they did require a lot of care. I received seventy-five dollars for Cindy, so reckoned she had been a good investment, returning three times what I had paid for her.

As I was growing older myself, and wanting more aloneness in which to pray and meditate, I was also glad to have the land to myself again. I don't think a day ever went by when I didn't spend at least an hour or two in the hollow or on the hillsides communing with God and nature, unless of course the weather was very cold or inclement. What I experienced there, listening to the wind in the top of the poplar trees or watching the ripples on the pond made by a solitary turtle paddling from one side to the other, must have made me a lover of Wordsworth, because when I first read "Lines Written a Few Miles Above Tintern Abbey" and "Ode on Intimations of Immortality" I knew exactly what he was talking about. As he said in "Tintern Abbey," "Nature never did betray the heart that loved her." There was a fullness there, of which I became a part, that quieted my heart at the same time that it excited it, and that has never deserted me.

It was during this period of my youth that I began to contemplate the ministry and eventually surrendered to it as a calling from God. I felt a growing calling among the rocks on that hillside, sitting there praying and experiencing a presence I couldn't explain apart from the divine. My thoughts weren't all sublime in those days; I moved through puberty into adolescence, and my blood was as normal as any teenage boy's. But that didn't stop me from enjoying flights of spirituality, a sense of transcendence that often overwhelmed me with feelings of both humility and invincibility.

I could return from worldly encounters, whether at school or at work, and be instantly transported into a kind of heavenly bliss. Never was I closer to the earth, and never closer to paradise.

$$\backsim$$

It was in this time too that I had my inexplicable encounter with the angel Gabriel. Like the call to the ministry, it was something I didn't solicit, something that merely happened. Yet there was no "merely" about it; it made a profound effect on my life and consciousness. It occurred one night in my little attic bedroom while I was on my knees in prayer. Suddenly I was aware of another presence in the room. There it was, a few feet away from me, a spectral being as tall as the low-ceilinged room itself. The light appeared to come from inside him, so that he was transparent, yet entirely visible. His features were elongated, like the paintings of El Greco's saints. I particularly remember that his hands were long and slender.

I did not have to be told that it was Gabriel; I knew it instinctively. And he didn't utter a single word. Just stood there, silently and majestically, for however long it was. I couldn't tell how long. Like all spiritual experiences, it was removed from the ordinary quantifications of time and space. I was breathless, I believe. I didn't say anything either. Then he was gone, and I felt both ecstasy and relief. I knew something important had happened, but I didn't know what. I wouldn't know, for a long time.

When I did figure it out, it was obvious. The appearance had been an extraordinary gift. I had seen what I had seen in order to give me an anchor for life, a fixed reference point that could not be shaken by anything I might encounter in my search for worldly or spiritual understanding.

I have never had any trouble believing that what I saw was real. First, it came unbidden. I had not been thinking about angels and didn't even particularly care about angels. I did not conjure this up out of my own imagination. Second, it didn't speak. If I had wanted this meeting, had sought it even in my unconscious, it would have spoken to me. I would have come away with some articulated message. Third, it was Gabriel and not Christ. If I had sown the seeds of this encounter in my subliminal self, I would have sought a vision of Jesus, who was much more on my mind those days. For years, in fact, I assumed it was an inferior vision because it didn't speak and wasn't of Jesus. And, fourth, I have never had any difficulty, at any time or in any place, conjuring up the effect of the vision all over again and knowing, without hesitance or doubt, that it was a valid appearance. There are some things one knows and knows one knows, and this was one of those. It was as real to me, and remains as real, as any meeting I ever had in my life. I will go as far as to say it was even more real. If everything that ever happened to me, every relationship and every encounter, were to dissolve today, this one would remain. It happened, and its happening had an eternal dimension and an eternal consequence.

Day after day and week after week, in my country retreat among the rocks and woods and hills, I fed upon that vision — pondered it, questioned it, prayed about it. And through all that time it nourished me, fed me deeply, as did the scene itself. Reality to me then became whatever I was experiencing in my soul, not what the world knew as reality, the routines and the commerce and the philosophies. I have used the word "invincibility." I did feel invincible now, in some strange way. Not that I couldn't be hurt or destroyed, for I could. But as if it didn't matter what happened to me, because God was so intimately present to my existence that nothing else counted. And it has been that way, more or less, for the remainder of my life.

Years later, when I was undergoing a spiritual upheaval and trying to decide whether to leave my teaching career at Vanderbilt to assume a pastorate, I had another encounter with Gabriel, albeit in a slightly different way. I was lying on the sofa in our den, practicing prayer and relaxation techniques while Anne was preparing dinner. The technique was to imagine a place where I felt great serenity and then simply permit a scene to occur —

to let the whole thing happen on its own without trying to manage it in the least.

The place was easy: I imagined myself on the hill above the peaceful little harbor on the Greek island of Paros where my son Eric and I had stayed in a hotel a few years before. It was a beautiful harbor, with water so clear and smooth on most days that one could actually see the shadows of boats on the bottom of the sea.

Suddenly there was movement and, totally without my willing it, a scenario began to unfold. An ancient galleon came sailing into the harbor — one of those old Spanish ships of the main from the days of the Great Armada. As it pulled into the dock I found myself running down the hill to greet it, with no clear purpose in mind, aware only that I must be there. I arrived at the dock just as the gangplank was laid down and the captain began to descend from the main deck. He was a regal figure in golden armor, and walked with magnificent authority.

Standing at the bottom of the gangplank, I awaited his arrival. He lifted the visor as he descended, then removed the helmet itself. With the visor up, he looked like the figure in Rembrandt's painting "The Man in the Golden Helmet." And then I realized who he was: it was Gabriel, the same figure I had seen all those years ago in my little attic bedroom!

"Don't you realize," he said, "that I have always been with you?"

And that was all. Like the spectral being in my bedroom, when it simply vanished, the waking dream was over. But in its place my soul was flooded by incredible peace and serenity. I knew I could make my decision about the pastorate and everything would be all right. This time I could believe that the apparition was summoned out of my own unconscious and its need for direction. But it was no less valid for that. Coupled with the initial occasion, when I had in no way bidden the presence, it was enormously consoling and encouraging. And again, as before, I can reconstitute the whole experience today by merely thinking about it, and it is just as real and effective as it was that evening in our den.

My first vision of Gabriel is the reason I always draw such strength from being in a beautiful natural setting. It is as if I am transported back again to that time and place on the little farm in Kentucky, and the presence is as real as ever. I feel, from the many hours of solitude in my small rural paradise, sensing the presence of the divine, that I have truly seen into the heart of things. It has made an enormous difference in my entire existence. All those years in libraries, in the halls of universities, in the pulpits and offices of churches, meeting people from literally every walk of life, were conditioned upon the time I enjoyed alone on those rocks and near that small body of water. And even now, as I lay down the mantle of responsibility and accept retirement, I sense that my attitude is entirely formed by what I experienced then and still believe to be the True North of my spiritual life.

☙

I have been many places and done many things since those formative years. Yet none of the places has ever replaced the one I knew then, or what I learned there.

I remember longing for it when I went off to Baylor University in Texas and had around me only flat, sandy soil with a few blades of grass and a smattering of live oaks and pecan trees. The only consolation there was the vast night sky, when the constellations of stars seemed so near that I could almost reach up and gather them the way one gathers apples off the low-hanging branches of a tree. I roomed in a big old house on South Fifth Street that we named the Robert E. Lee Mansion, a house as graceless as the nondescript fellows who lived there. But at night I could go out onto the flat roof behind my room, lie there on the warm tarpaper, and look up into the endless sky and hovering stars, and feel that overwhelming presence again.

I grew away from my hillside retreat during that first autumn in Waco, Texas, and it was never again the same to me. But I can still recall the excitement I felt driving home at Christmas, when I saw the increasing greenness of the land and the reappearance of the great oaks and maples whose grandeur had always thrilled me. I could not believe how green the grass appeared, even in winter, compared with the brownscapes of Texas, or how beautiful the hills were, especially in Tennessee and Kentucky, after the barrenness of Waco and Dallas.

Even when I did get back home after that, I was busy working on my college degree, marrying, and then attending graduate school, and simply didn't have time to wander over the hills and along the creeks as I once did. But as Wordsworth said, there are still "sensations sweet" that are "felt in the blood." Even today, years after my parents died and I sold the old home place because I couldn't care for it from a distance, those early times spent in that cradle of the spirit continue to speak to my heart with more cogency than any place I've ever known.

⌁

It was while I was still a young man walking those hills and sitting among those rocks that I discovered the great romance of books. The wonder and mystery I had loved in nature grew even deeper in books. The Bible came first, of course, and was the first real book I ever owned. I began reading it in earnest after I became a Christian at the age of eleven. For years I would not put a mark in it because I regarded it as too holy for that kind of desecration. Then, when I was fifteen and a junior in high school writing weekly themes for a demanding English and Latin teacher named Jeanne Fightmaster (behind her back, we called her Miss Pugnomagister, the Latin equivalent of her name), I fell in love with words and began devouring the dictionary my parents had given me as a birthday present. I also bought two books by Wilfred Funk, the renowned verbologist, on the power of language, and read them avidly too.

It was at this time that I began purchasing the books that attracted me to the world of humane letters. First was Anderson M. Baten's *The Philosophy of Life,* a delightful compendium of paragraphs, poems, epigrams, and essays by many of the world's greatest writers from Plato to Shakespeare and Milton to Montaigne. Many of the selections were sentimental favorites, such as Rudyard Kipling's "L'Envoi" ("When Earth's last picture is painted, and the tubes are twisted and dried") and William Ernest Henley's "Invictus" ("Out of the night that covers me,/ Black as the pit from pole to pole"), and I read them so often that their words sang in my heart even when I wasn't directly thinking about them. Then came Will and Ariel Durant's *The Story of Philosophy,* that sweeping, majestic summary from the authors' life's work among the great thinkers of the world, written in the kind of beautiful, limpid prose some of the philosophers themselves never mastered. I wandered in and out among the thoughts that helped shape our civilization, and was enchanted by these mental contacts with a universe so much grander than the small, semirural one I had known.

During my senior year in high school, the Garden City Publishing Company of Garden City, New York, began issuing its magnificent series of Perma Giants by Henry and Dana Lee Thomas. At ninety-five cents each, they were handsomely designed and sturdily assembled volumes of Living Biographies of the great poets, artists, novelists, philosophers, scientists, composers, and religious leaders. Every life was treated with admiration and enthusiasm, and the writing was of the pellucid, upbeat style once employed in the *Reader's Digest.* I acquired every volume I ever saw, and still have them on my shelves today. And even now, when I occasionally revisit them, I find them highly inspirational.

I regret that my parents were not readers (my father did enjoy Westerns and murder mysteries) and did not encourage me to read the great novels of the world, the way my wife's mother did her. My father owned a glass-fronted bookcase that contained on one shelf a row of leather-bound Harvard Classics — they had come with the bookcase — but he did not like for anyone to touch them. After he died I let them go with the furnishings to a secondhand dealer, thinking it a pity that they had been forbidden to me as a boy and that I no longer wanted them, now that I owned them in other, more readable editions. But untutored as I was, I confess that at that time I still thought of fiction as less than serious in a world where there was so much to master in the realms of pure knowledge.

There was a great Scottish minister — perhaps it was Alexander Whyte — who used to advise his students at the university to sell their beds, if they must, in order to buy books. For years, I didn't even have a bed to sell, and thus could afford only a few books that I carefully and lovingly selected. Even at Harvard, after I had already earned a Ph.D. in literature, I hadn't the money to purchase all the textbooks required in my courses, so spent a lot of time in the library reading and making notes. But I was overjoyed to learn, when we moved to the Boston area, how many wonderful used-bookstores there were, where volumes were much more affordable. And when I was called to the little church I pastored during my Harvard days, on the south edge of Andover, Massachusetts, I could hardly believe my good fortune at discovering a small used-bookstore a few hundred yards from the parsonage.

It was in an old building that probably once housed a neighborhood grocery store or a small filling station, and that had now been painted forest green with white trim around the door and windows. It was owned and managed by a short, bald, comical-looking little man who had once been a truck driver and still spoke like one. But he loved books, especially old books from the broken libraries of the deceased, and he had literally crammed that small building with every kind of book one could imagine. Every week I spent an hour or two poking around to see what new treasures he had found. I still have dozens of volumes from that tiny store — Thomas Carlyle, John Ruskin, Phillips Brooks, George Bernard Shaw, and others — most of which cost only a quarter.

The thing about books, for me, is that they are the doorways to so many wonderful minds and places, vehicles for broadening oneself and becoming acquainted with the world. In this way they are part of the mystery and miracle I discerned in the world from the beginning, and represent only an expansion of the spirit of divine intrigue I felt in the universe when I was a small boy.

The books that have come into my hands across the years have introduced me to a great deal of life and thought that might otherwise have
remained inaccessible to me. And if I have often been judged to be radical,
unorthodox, or too adventurous in my own ideas, it is probably because I
have such a deep respect for the variety of minds and experiences I have
encountered in my reading. It is hard to remain parochial and exclusivist
in one's religious and political ideologies when one is accustomed to entertaining the thoughts and images of many wonderful writers in other
faiths and traditions and other parts of the globe. For me, much of the
beauty and mystery of God's universe stems from the enormous variety
of people, things, and experiences that are crammed into it, and I revel
in all of that as I once delighted in the woods and creeks of my boyhood
Kentucky.

☙

The linchpin of my adult life, if there is one, was surely the fifteen years
when I was a professor at Vanderbilt University. I had never intended
during the period of my training to become a professor, but they say that
life is what happens when you are expecting something else and that was
indeed the case for me.

Those were years of great joy and enormous growth when, for the first
time, I had not only the leisure to think and write about almost anything
I chose but also a great deal of unclaimed time to spend with my lovely
wife and our two growing sons. Teaching in religion and the humanities
has never paid well monetarily, but it is rich in other gifts, such as the
chance to associate with the well-educated and the opportunity to spend
expanses of time with one's family. I once calculated, considering the long
holidays and extensive summer vacations we were given at Vanderbilt,
that I worked only seven months a year, and then only on two or three
days of the week. I was almost invariably home — except for speaking and
lecture trips — when our sons came in from school, and always had time

for a game of football or basketball, or merely to sit while they had their snacks and listen to their tales of the day.

Add to that the three sabbaticals I had during my tenure at Vanderbilt, plus the hundreds if not thousands of speaking trips I was privileged to make — some to such exotic locations as Berchtesgarten, Austria; Chichicastenango, Guatemala; and Bangkok, Thailand — and it will be obvious that our years in Nashville were a fascinating time of expanding love and awareness, when the sense of mystery I experienced as a child now continued, more heartily than ever, as an exploration of people, places, and ideas.

We built a home in Nashville on a beautiful two-acre lot in the charming old section near Ensworth School and Montgomery Bell Academy, both of which our sons attended. It was not a conventional lot, for it was shaped like the end of a boomerang whose center was the home of Mr. George Knox, a banker, at the very end of Ensworth Avenue. Mr. Knox's son was in med school and needed money for his tuition. So he agreed to sell us the end of the boomerang, which didn't have a proper opening to any street although it was separated only by a drainage ditch from a small, intimate circle on Clearview Drive, a much less prestigious street than Ensworth. Prestige meant nothing to us, but beauty and accessibility did, so we bought the lot and cut a small opening from one corner of it into that circle on Clearview Drive. Thus our property was mostly hidden from the street and approached through a little bower of trees, and we always felt that it was a beautiful haven from the world outside.

There we laughed and loved and celebrated life, even creating new holidays for the months when there were no special ones. If I had set out in the beginning to construct an idyllic existence, I can't imagine that I could have done any better than the life we enjoyed. It had its minor ups and downs, of course. But on the whole it remains in my memory as a long, extended period of bliss and happiness, when our problems were small and our blessings incredibly great. Our very existence in those years, as I recall them, seemed sacramental, as if it were always verging on the special and the holy.

I remember the beautiful Christmas eve in 1968, the year we returned from our enchanting sojourn in Paris. We had all agreed — we consulted our sons as if they were young adults — to attend the midnight service at Vine Street Christian Church, a few blocks from our home. It was a lovely service. The music and sermon perfectly suited our spirits. And when the ushers began to pass the communion plates, Eric, our seven-year-old, whispered to me that he would like to take his first communion. Surprised, I asked if he understood what it was about. He said he did. I leaned over and whispered to Anne that our son wanted to receive communion too. Was it all right with her? She smiled and nodded. With his head bowed and the nape of his neck peeking out over his collar, he prayed over the bread and then the cup, and received his first communion.

When we came out, the church bells were ringing wildly above us and big, heavy snowflakes were falling all around us. We couldn't imagine a finer Christmas gift or a happier time.

When I mentioned the nape of Eric's neck, it reminded me of something I read once in a book by François Mauriac, who said that in his latter years he could not bear to go to low mass any more because he felt so sublimely unnerved by the napes of the children's necks as they bent in prayer. He was right. It is one of the most beautiful and moving sights in the world.

A few years later, both our sons were baptized by our minister at the Second Presbyterian Church, the Rev. Mr. Joseph Holder. Anne and I never pushed our sons toward our own religion but were happy when they elected it on their own. I remember shopping for half a day on the Saturday before Krister was baptized to find just the right little silver cross as a memento of the occasion, and Anne and I wrote a special hymn that was sung by the alto soloist that Sunday.

It was a haunting mixture of beauty and pathos, for I was beginning to have presentiments about the time when we would not be able to shelter our children as we did then. It was called "He Was a Lamb," and was set in a minor key.

> He was a Lamb
> Born in a world of wolves,
> And the wolves began to howl
> When he was born.
> What is it makes us hate the innocent?
> What makes us restless
> Till its heart is torn?
> A little Lamb,
> A little Lamb,
> And we hated him
> For even being born.

Perhaps the sense of pathos arose from my own growing unsettledness and the feeling that our world was about to change. For in 1976, when the Plymouth Congregational Church in Minneapolis offered me a position as its minister, I began to experience low rumblings — like the beginnings of an earthquake — in my thoughts about the future, and by 1978 I was actively looking around the country to see where I might fit as some church's senior minister.

Even as I conducted my search, however, something inside me fought doggedly against going, for our time in Nashville had been the most beautiful, halcyon years any family ever had. There were moments when I went outside and walked around our house, staring at it and thinking, "I can't leave this place. This is the nearest to paradise we'll ever get in this life."

It took me two or three years, after going to the First Presbyterian Church of Lynchburg, Virginia, to get over longing to return to Nashville and reoccupy our beautiful home on Clearview Drive. It would always remain the benchmark by which I judged the other homes we lived in and the communities around them.

In the pastorate, I pursued the sense of mystery and divine intrigue with more deliberateness and intensity than I ever had in the past. There, both in Lynchburg and later in Los Angeles, the focus was on people, lots of people, and many of them had some kind of personal problem, some grievance, some attitude that was tearing up their lives or the lives of the people around them. I had always loved people, and in my pastorates I found that I loved them even more than before.

Often it was the odd or different ones I liked best. Horsley Putt, the big, hulking old softie of a man who lived as a kind of minor con artist, always with huge plans and usually wanting to involve his pastor in them, but essentially always in need of money because he wasn't very successful in his career as a salesman and lived above his means. Deanne Gwaltney, the funny little old lady who was obsequiously twittering when I went to call on her, and behaved so deferentially that I sometimes wanted to shake her and remind her that I was only a human being like herself. Tex McCoy, the pencil-thin, toothless old cowboy who needed a shave and liked to dance a little jig in the forecourt outside our church in Los Angeles. Esther Dunnigan, the elegant transvestite who looked so beautiful in her expensive clothes and heels that half the men in the congregation turned to stare at her until they realized she had a mustache. Then they stared again.

These were God's children, maybe even his best people. Being their pastor made me happy with ministry. I felt as if I belonged somewhere, and we were all going to heaven together. A lot of people in my churches resented the time I spent on the outcasts and ne'er-do-wells, but I loved them, and they people my memories of the pastorate with a kind of panache the other, more ordinary folks didn't give it.

It was in them, and in the prayers I composed for my congregations, that I felt nearest to God in those days. Buttrick was right about spending time on the prayers. I didn't devote an inordinate amount of time — I was too busy to labor over them longer than necessary — but I never went into the chancel on Sunday morning without a feeling that I had done my best to achieve the phrasings and images that would help people to engage in their own prayers while I led them. If my prayers were evocative of love and serenity, it was because I felt those qualities in my heart and wanted them to abound in the world. Yet I also frequently prayed about the fragmented condition of the world, and what we could do to improve people's situations.

☙

Perhaps, more than anything else, the theme of my ministry in the churches I served was seeking union with the holy. I wanted everybody to enjoy the sense of oneness I myself felt with God, the mystical joy I had always known in him, but I knew that it was absent in so many people's lives. If I could only say or do something that would show them the glory they were missing, the delight they could be taking in one another, in the greater world community, in the created order, then I would be happy and feel fulfilled in my calling.

Alas, it is a vision difficult to convey to those who have not come to it on their own. If I wept over anything in particular in my ministry, it was my inability to reach most people, to open their eyes to the wonderful gifts God was able and willing to bestow upon them. Again and again I was shocked and disturbed by things said or done in board meetings of the church that struck me as being so obviously against the will and purpose of God. How could people who had sat through worship service after worship service with me remain so benighted about the love and the desire of God? Clearly I had failed to communicate to them the vision and serenity that filled my own soul.

Yet I knew a great peace in ministry, and was certain that I had done the right thing in giving up our beautiful home in Nashville to pursue the calling. I felt as if my life burned with the steady flame of a mature torch, consuming itself in the process, and that it was thus paying homage to the greatest ideal in the world, the presence of a loving, life-honoring God. If I lacked the time for personal mysticism and devotion that I had known as a youngster on the farm and then a professor in the university, I was making up for it in fidelity and service. That in itself made me feel close to God and gave me a sense of great satisfaction.

༄

When I finally left the pastoral ministry to return to teaching, part of the reason was my strong desire to have more time again, to be able to wander the world and pray without the weight of a large congregation on my back. I wasn't trying to be selfish. I merely needed to feel again the great sense of intimacy with the divine that had always been a part of my daily experience, and to do so without an overwhelming "to do" list crowding my consciousness.

I remember praying long and hard about whether I should resign my pastorate in Los Angeles to accept the offer that had come from Samford University in Birmingham. One day, as I knelt over an overstuffed chair in our living room, I imagined I heard God's answer to my desperate prayers.

"I want my little boy back again," he said.

Maybe it was an answer from God, and maybe it came from my own unconscious. But I knew what it meant. It meant that in spite of my dawn-to-dusk efforts to serve my parishes and make everything all right for everybody, I was spiritually starving as a pastor.

Probably few parishioners are ever struck by the spiritual poverty of their ministers, and yet it is almost a given in ministry. It is like the old saying that the cobbler's children never have shoes. Ministers are so busy tending to the spiritual life of their congregations that they usually have little time for their own. This was not always true, of course; only in modern times, with the diversification of parishes, the complexity of life in metropolitan areas, the extreme busyness of members, and the pressures under which they live, have churches become almost impossible challenges to the imagination and oversight of pastors.

When I reflect on whether God actually did get his little boy back again in Birmingham, I have to say only a qualified yes. Beyond a few

new friendships, I received almost nothing from the university that en-
hanced my sense of spirituality. But over the next several years, I strove to
rediscover that "little boy" and the wonder that he experienced so fully.

c∙ɔ

One luxury I gave myself after arriving in Birmingham was four months of
Jungian therapy with a remarkably perceptive analyst. Like most Jungians,
she preferred to work with her clients' dreams, for they tell so much of
what is happening on the inner scene. I soon became a "dream-catcher,"
awakening several times in the night to write down the scenario I had just
experienced.

At first, many of my dreams dealt with institutionalism and the difficulty
of finding myself in a welter of competing voices. Sometimes I would be
fleeing down a dark street or alley with arms reaching out of the shadows
to seize me. And not a few of my dreams involved having to clean up
filth and ordure — subject matter that the therapist assured me was not
unusual for ministers, who often have to deal with other people's messes.

Eventually, though, the dreams became pleasant and serene, signaling
my arrival at a new point in my feelings. And just before Easter that year,
near the end of my therapy, I dreamed that I had gone fishing in a lovely,
verdant area — it occurred to me that it was the original paradise — and
the water was apparently teeming with fish. I threw in my line — I was
using an old-fashioned cane pole and a hook baited with a worm — and
instantly caught a huge fish. Half the worm was still on the hook, so I
tossed it in again. Again, I caught a large fish. Now the hook was empty,
but things were going so well that I couldn't resist throwing it back into
the water. A third time, I caught an enormous fish. I had them lying there
on the bank, head-to-tail in a rough sort of triangle, and was amazed at
my good fortune.

When I narrated this dream for the therapist, she didn't say a word.
Instead, she got up, crossed the room, took down a large book from the
library shelves, and turned to a page she wanted me to see. It had a

drawing on it of three plump fish lying head-to-tail, as in my dream. And the caption beneath the drawing said: "An ancient symbol of Christianity and the kingdom of God; a sign of great fullness and joy."

Poring over the deep stack of pages containing the dreams of that pe-riod, I realize it is time for me to review them and see what they may have to reveal to me today. At the very least they are evidence of the great mysteries among which I live, and of the way my soul is enriched by the work being done all the time in my own unconscious, where I am not even aware of it.

c-ɔ

One of the things that came from my therapy was a chance to liaise in a more conscious way with my own anima, the female principle at the heart of my existence as a man. It was no accident, I think, that I soon after began writing my first Jessie novel, about a female Christ-figure, and found real spiritual satisfaction in doing that.

Interestingly, I set that novel in the area around Gatlinburg, Tennessee, where Jessie could reflect my own enjoyment of the exquisite scenery and great hiking trails of the Smoky Mountains. One of the highest moments of the story occurs when Jessie and her friends Roxie, Joan, and Phyllis, with Jessie's dog, Columbo, climb up Chimney Tops, one of the great peaks of the Smokies, and basically reenact the scene between Jesus and his disciples on the Mount of Transfiguration. Passing little mountain streams frolicking in the sunlight and small dells riotous with wild flowers, they finally sit to rest a while at the top of the mountain: "A hawk descended from somewhere in a narrowing spiral and landed on a dead tree branch on a little knoll a dozen yards away. Columbo, aware of the circling shadow, pricked his ears and raised his head to see the landing, then lowered it again.

"Joan, who had taken repose against a tree a few feet from Jessie, was watching her face in love and admiration. For a moment, the sun in its westward travels dipped behind a cloud, which cast a slight shadow over the spot where Jessie sat. Then, reaching the edge of the cloud, the sun shone fully in her face, causing her to close her eyes and tilt her chin up until the rays transformed the planes of her cheeks into pools of light.

"Joan's mouth dropped partly open, and she started, unable to breathe for a few seconds. It was as if heaven itself were anointing her dear friend Jessie, whose being, she had always believed, was the purest and most angelic the world had ever known.

"The hawk sailed into the air again, breaking the spell of the moment. But Joan knew she would never forget what she had witnessed.

"Presently Roxie came out of her resting place among the trees and stood, hands on hips, surveying the wideness of peaks and valleys.

" 'God,' she said, 'this really is the most fantastic place. Don't you think we could just stay up here, Jess, and never go down?' "

This was my vintage life, as it has always been. By the grace of God, my "little boy" had survived the years of university and parish life, and was once again flourishing. I'm happy to say he's alive and well today.

Do I still feel what I did in those earliest years, a sense of the mystery of God inhabiting everything in the world? Indeed I do. If anything, the feeling is stronger than ever, now that I have time to attend to it every day. Work is wonderful, and I wouldn't take anything for my experiences of it throughout my lifetime. But as I said in the chapter on working, it does sometimes act as a screen that prevents us from seeing the presence of the holy as directly as we might otherwise behold it. Now I get up in the morning with no compulsion to do this or that during the day and feel that I am essentially back where I was when I was a boy on that wonderful little farm in Kentucky. The world is a gift to open, and God is standing there waiting to see how I like it.

Ten

A Feast of Coalescence

A few months ago, I lay in a hospital bed in Saint Joseph Mercy Hospital in Detroit, Michigan. I had had surgery to remove a mysterious spot that appeared on the upper lobe of my right lung. The surgery had gone as expected and I had been doing so well that I was sent directly to an ordinary hospital room, not to ICU. A couple of days later I was up, dragging my IV-stand and strolling the halls. Then, four days after surgery, I bent over to pick up a pillow that had fallen on the floor and suddenly felt breathless and nauseated. My wonderful new Indian friend, Dr. Amit Dwiveda, came to see me a few moments later, realized what was happening, and ordered emergency procedures. My body had sent a shower of emboli into the wound in my lung.

The day became a series of activities bent on saving my life. I was moved immediately into ICU and given intravenous Heparin, a strong blood thinner. My dear friends, Dr. and Mrs. Yvan Silva, who lived in Detroit and were members of our Mackinac Island parish, sat in my room for an hour or more while another doctor moved a sonar scanner back and forth over my legs, searching for more clots and trying to determine where the first ones had originated.

Yvan wasn't on duty, as it was Sunday. When he and Marcie left, he took my head in his hands and kissed my forehead. I was very touched.

The Heparin was discontinued and shortly after that I was wheeled away to an operating room where a doctor inserted a Greenfield filter through my groin into the *vena cava*, or primary vein running from the legs to the heart, so that if I shot any more clots they would be held in transit while my immune system dissolved them. Then the Heparin infusions were started again.

My wife, Anne, our son Eric, and his recent bride, Pia, were in Detroit with me and spent an anxious day while all this was transpiring. The doctors had alerted us to the danger. There was a more than fifty-fifty chance that the onset of the clots that morning should have killed me, they said. But I would not be out of the woods for some time. Visiting hours in ICU were over at eight. I hugged Anne, Eric, and Pia as they left for their motel, and told Anne to call our son Kris in Virginia and alert him to the possibilities of what could happen.

On their way out of the hospital, Anne asked Eric and Pia if they could stop for a few minutes in the chapel to pray. They knelt along a kneeling rail at the back of the room and prayed silently in the soft candlelight.

Then the most extraordinary thing occurred.

Anne had been praying and crying. She looked up and was staring through her tears at the beautiful wooden reredos featuring the stations of the cross. Suddenly a spirit thing — a white, gauzy shape the size of a man — spun out of the reredos, drifted up the aisle past her and the others, and out the doors in the back of the chapel. She saw it first out of the corner of her eye, and remembered that an ophthalmologist had said she had the beginnings of a cataract. Then she looked straight at it, and knew it wasn't an optical illusion.

Suspecting that she might be hallucinating, she turned to Eric, who was praying beside her, and saw that his eyes were open and he was staring ahead.

"Eric," she said quietly, "did you see anything just now?"

"Yes."

"What was it?"

"Something white. It billowed out of the reredos and went up the aisle past us."

It was one of those incredible moments that become all the more real because they are so unreal that they stand out from the others. Pia, the third person present in the chapel, did not see what the others saw. But the important thing was that both Anne and Eric saw it. And neither of them is given to mystical experiences or flights of fancy.

Eric was in the final year of his studies for a Ph.D. in depth psychology at Pacifica Graduate Institute in California. He wrote a paper about the experience for a course in numinology. It was clearly a numinous revelation, he said — a divine visitation in a visible form. He and his mother had actually seen something supernatural!

Anne's first thought, after she realized what they had seen, was "Gabriel!" She knew my experiences with the angel, and assumed this must be his way of saying, "It's okay, he will recover." Suddenly, she said, a great calm fell over her spirit, which until that moment had been deeply agitated. She was able to return to the motel, call Kris, go to bed and sleep peacefully, knowing that I would be all right.

I am glad she made this connection, for it is the one I myself would have made. If I had died, I might have beheld Gabriel myself. But, as I didn't, I received Anne and Eric's report as a divine confirmation of the segment of life on which I am now embarked — the years of retirement when I am freer to pursue the spiritual dimension of existence than I have ever been in my life.

And what I have noticed — the thing that makes this time of life so delightful — is the way all the strands of my being that have thus far appeared to be separate and individual are beginning to come together to form a whole. They probably never were as distinct as I imagined them to be. But now they are converging in a way that is almost breathtaking.

There is a principle in physics known as the Casimir effect, named for the Dutch physicist who first described it. It is the principle that if two plates are brought close to one another, the vacuum of energy between them will force them together. The classic analogy of the principle is of two schooners drawing so close to one another on the high seas that they inevitably collide. What happens is that the waves between the ships, because the ships form their boundaries, are all of the same size and are shorter and less powerful than the waves on the outer sides of the ships. Therefore the waves on the outer sides actually push the ships together.

Perhaps, as we grow older, the Casimir effect occurs in our lives. The re-lationships among all the tracks of our existence are so close that the forces outside us inevitably make it appear that they are being compelled into unity. Or maybe it was only an illusion that they were ever that separate and distinct to begin with. Possibly, if we were wiser and more sensitive from our youth, we would perceive their nearness and the inevitability that they would one day collide.

I am inclined to believe, from the vantage point of age, that the latter is really the case and the strands of our existence are always much nearer to one another than we ever suspect. When we grow older, especially after we have retired and possess the leisure to feel and observe things with patience and clarity, we experience the unification of all these strands as a truly spiritual occurrence. God has been in them all along, but now we are amazed to discover that fact and the discovery itself is like a revelation.

ᕲ

To begin with, we have all this time to remember things — all the wonder-ful places we've ever visited and the beautiful people we have known. It is commonly said that old age is a time of forgetfulness. Don't believe it! Sometimes the synapses are a little sluggish — maybe they too are subject to arthritis — but they always get there eventually. And our memories are better than ever for the things that matter most, such as culling through the mental files of our childhoods and young-adult years for the delightful events and images that have contributed so much toward making us who we are today. As I said in the first chapter of this book, our latter years are haunted!

If I spin the memory wheel now, for example, the first thing the pointer lands on, without any effort on my part, is an image of Gerard Simonnot, a tall, distinguished-looking friend we acquired the year we lived in Paris. Gerry was married to Georgie, a woman more than twenty years his senior, and he once told us why. His mother was English and his father was French. After his father died, his mother moved to Paris and opened a milliner's shop with Georgie, who had been a friend of the family. Gerry was about fifteen at the time, and of course moved to Paris with his mother. A couple of years later his mother met and married another gentleman, and they went off on their honeymoon, leaving Georgie in charge of Gerry. While they were gone Georgie seduced the young boy, hustled him off to the registry office, and married him. His mother had a conniption fit about it when she returned, but there was nothing she could do. Gerry was sweet on Anne, and corresponded with us for years after we left Paris. When Georgie died he married again — this time, he said, for love.

Another spin, and this time the pointer stops on a childhood memory when I was four or five. I was in the side yard of our little home in Stanford, Kentucky, with a mini-sized baseball bat in my hand. I had been hitting an old rubber ball around the yard. A blue jay landed on the corner of my little sandbox. Impulsively, I hurled the bat end-over-end at the bird, striking and killing it. I was devastated, and thought I would surely be punished by some divine hand for such a terrible deed. I went into the house and got a wooden strawberry carton, took it outside, put some grass in the bottom, and gently laid the bird on the grass. Digging a hole in the back garden, I placed the carton in it and covered everything with dirt. I hoped that God, or whoever was in charge of the lives of birds, would have mercy on me. It would be hard, I knew, because I was having trouble forgiving myself.

Yet again. This time I am a nine-year-old in Cynthiana, Kentucky, playing tackle football with a gang of boys in the back yard of John Swinford, the young man who lived across the street from us. John's dad was a federal judge, and they had a big home with a large yard, so we usually played there. It was cold and rainy, and the earth was muddy. I can remember the smell of the dampness and the mold. I had recently acquired my first pair of glasses, but I wasn't wearing them to play football, so I didn't see things as clearly as I wanted to. There was a lot of confusion in the action, with boys running into one another and piling on the one who was caught with the ball. I didn't like all the physical contact and the messiness of playing in the mud. But I played hard in spite of that, because I was fast and enjoyed the exhilarating experience of trying to elude the other players.

Once more. I remember Sam Flynn, a poor farmer in my first parish, in Bronston, Kentucky. And when I remember Sam, I see his beautiful little blond wife, Roberta, and their sweet, well-mannered children, three or four under the age of five. The Flynns were extremely poor because their farm was tiny and no matter how hard they worked there were never enough crops or cattle. They all looked thin and undernourished, with shining eyes that almost popped out of their faces, like the people in photographs from the drought-tortured areas of Africa. But they were enormously kind, adoring people, and their children were shy and well behaved. And they clearly loved one another with great intensity. When we went to their home for a meal we tried not to eat much because we knew their food was scarce.

I could do this all day and all night. In fact, a lot of the time it is what I do. All the portraits, all the events, keep flooding the screen without ceasing. Yet they appear to be inexhaustible, as if I could spend the remainder of my years watching and listening to them and still not see all of them. It is as if I had direct TV with a thousand stations, and they are all transmitting to my screen at the same time.

I am grateful for the memories, and thank God every day for them, for they are the substance of my life. Not the sum of it, but the substance. They are what has happened in my conscious existence, and therefore they account for much of who I am today.

৻৲

But memories are not everything. I am also grateful for my body, which continues, in spite of the surgery and the blood clots, to be a happy residence for my spirit. I read a statement in the *Washington Post*, in a re-view of Alice Flaherty's *The Midnight Disease: The Drive to Write, Writer's Block, and the Creative Brain,* that "All the works of the spirit are made with corrupt bodies." I understand what she meant, but think she over-stated the case. I'm not comfortable with the old medieval attitude toward the body. Frankly I like my body and do not think of it as corrupt. It has served me well and I am very pleased with it.

Today, I went to my exercise club at noon and worked out for an hour. I try to go at least three times a week. While I'm walking up a stiff incline on the treadmill at four miles an hour or doing a hundred and fifty sit-ups on a tummy-buster or bench-pressing a hundred pounds for seventy repetitions, my spirit contemplates all kinds of things, and feels an amazing closeness to God. I realized this as I worked out today. I thought, "I am sensing the presence of God here as much as I ever do in church listening to a big choir or hearing a good sermon. God is somehow in my body and this workout."

I was being grateful for the body I've been allowed to live in all these years. It made me remember one time in Colorado when I became so excited about life that I embarrassed our young sons. We had been to Waco, Texas, where I spoke to the board of Word Publishing Company. When I finished, I mentioned to Jarrell McCracken, Word's president, that we had a tent in the back of our station wagon and were on our way to Colorado for some camping. Jarrell reached in his pocket, took out a key, and dangled it in front of me.

"Wouldn't you prefer to sleep in a cabin?" he asked.

It wasn't a very pretentious cabin, Jarrell warned us, and there might not be many other people in the area because it was early June and most of the cabin-owners didn't arrive until July or August. He was right about that. I don't think we saw another soul in the Sangre de Cristo Mountains. But the cabin was fantastic! It was large and comfortable and looked as if it had been decorated by a New York designer. And there was a little trout stream gurgling down the mountain right beside it.

One day Anne, the boys, and I went for a hike into the nearby mountains. After climbing for an hour or more, we came to a ridgetop, and followed a trail through some woods and rock formations. I was enjoying the exercise so much that I was a couple of hundred yards ahead of the boys, and Anne was bringing up the rear. So I was the first to come upon a simply unbelievable meadow way up in the mountains — a wide space of flat land brimming with daisies and columbines, where bees and butterflies were working their little butts off pollinating everything.

I couldn't help myself. Such a vision called for extreme measures. Removing all my clothes — every stitch of them — I pranced and frolicked across that meadow as if I were cavorting in a dream. It was glorious! I had to be in paradise!

But then I heard Kris, our youngest, hollering from the edge of the woods, "Mom! Come quick! Dad's gone crazy!"

The boys still laugh about that. And I remember the ecstasy of it as if it happened only a few hours ago. It was wonderful. I am proud of my spontaneity for doing it. It was one of the few truly spontaneous responses of that sort I ever made, and the fact that I did it is one of the golden trophies in my mind. I was truly *in* my body.

I admit that pain and illness are problems with the body, especially as we grow older. But maybe they are reminders of the fact that our bodies won't go on forever, or, for that matter, our personalities as we now recognize them. I know, when I have the flu or am experiencing a touch of phlebitis, as I did after my lung surgery, that the time will come when I am thoroughly ready to give up this body and leave my earthly existence. As a pastor, I have known many older parishioners who complained that they were actually tired of their bodies and wanted to be released from them. I expect that time to come for me. But by then I hope I will have brought the loose ends of myself together in such a way that I feel completely orderly in my spirit, and that everything about me has coalesced in such a way as to pronounce me whole and ready to die.

I like something in Browning Ware's *Diary of a Modern Pilgrim.* Ware
had asked his friend Buckner Fanning about a recent illness. "You know,
Browning," quipped Fanning, "I think God is calling me home on the
installment plan."[7]

Maybe that's the way it works, and we'll all be ready to go when the
final payment is due. But things are coming together — memories, body,
friends and associates....

⁓

I used to worry that Anne and I had moved around so much that we no
longer knew where home was and didn't really have a community of the
kind many people enjoy. It is ironic, but a minister lives most of his or her
life with a kind of instant community, then retires and doesn't have one.
We thought once about going back to the town in Kentucky where we
met and married, but decided that wouldn't work because it is no longer
the town we once knew. The beautiful little town square, once the center
of life in the community, is no longer the center. A highway bypassing
the town long ago became the primary commercial area, drawing off most
of the businesses that once made the square so vital. When we go back
now we are almost overwhelmed by the crowds of people in the shopping
centers, and wonder where they've come from. Certainly it wasn't that
way when we lived there. Our old church isn't the same any more. And
most of the people we once knew are either dead and gone or have become
somebody else over the years.

We have flirted with the idea of moving to Florida or California, where
we would be warm in the winter, but then we realize that we actually like
the snow and cold weather. We would miss it if we didn't have it, especially
in the evening when we enjoy a big wood fire in the grate as we read, talk,
or watch a movie. We live in an area thick with history — battlegrounds
and old houses and historic buildings — and can always find something
to amuse ourselves when we want to, with day trips and luncheons in
favorite little pubs or tearooms. We also live very close to both of our sons

and their wives, and to our grandchildren, Ellie and Chloe. If we went off to an artificial community somewhere, we wouldn't see them very often.

What we do have now is an e-community — hosts of friends all over the United States and the world who in one sense are no farther away from us than the computer screen. E-mail is a wonderful boon. It brings our friends into intimate range wherever they are. Many of them carry their laptops with them on vacation, and whether they're in St. Petersburg, Paris, or Acapulco, they still keep in touch.

Opening the e-mail every day is even more fun than going to the mail box used to be because we get far more mail this way than we ever did by conventional mail. On any given day I'm likely to hear from friends in New York, New Jersey, Florida, Alabama, Tennessee, North Carolina, Nebraska, Indiana, Illinois, Michigan, California, Texas, and any of a dozen other states, as well as two or three countries overseas.

Anne also hears from many friends, and often forwards their messages to my machine so I'll see them too. Many of the people who correspond with her send forwarded pieces, mostly humorous in nature, and she acts as my screen, sending on the ones she thinks I'll enjoy and deleting the others. And we both forward our share of funny stories and epigrams to our children and other friends.

Another delight of electronic mail is hearing frequently from people who begin by saying, "You don't know me, but I read your book" or "You probably won't remember me, but I heard you speak at this or that meeting a dozen years ago." I always answer messages from people who have gone to the trouble to track me down and send a letter, because it is a genuine pleasure to hear from them. In my lifetime I have written to perhaps a dozen authors about their works, always adulatory letters because I found their books so entrancing, and have received responses from only one or two. So I try to raise the average by being as thoughtful and generous to writers as I possibly can.

The thing is, as I suggested, this e-community is very important in a world where the older kinds of community have largely broken down. We see very little of our neighbors in the subdivision where we live. Most of them are working couples with teenage children, and we know from their comings and goings how little time they have for collegiality with their neighbors. But I sit up in my study, which overlooks most of the other houses in the neighborhood for a view of the mountains beyond, and peck away messages to friends around the world, and they write back to me. We can't reach out and touch one another literally, the way neighbors used to do, but at least we send our thoughts and feelings back and forth, and it's the next best thing. I imagine that even a person in prison who has access to a computer and the Internet can still feel connected to the rest of the world, and not isolated the way prisoners always were in the past.

જ્જ

Everything is coming together — even my greatest concerns.

What is my principal worry as I grow older? It's the enormous trouble our world is in, and the nearly unimaginable suffering of so many millions of people. I pray every day for the masses of persons who are hungry, ill, broken, or abused, and for all those who are grieving for loved ones who have been killed or imprisoned. When that terrible earthquake occurred in Bam, Iran, taking more than thirty thousand lives, and a powerful tsunami devastated the nations around the Indian Ocean, destroying hundreds of thousands, I prayed for months for their souls and for the survivors whose lives were so rudely transformed by the loss of people they loved. My head couldn't get around the magnitude of such events, and I had a helpless feeling as I tried to pray for all those poor families. It was like trying to empty the ocean with an eyedropper. Similarly my heart has ached for the thousands and thousands of people affected by the war in Iraq and the senseless bombings and killings in Israel, Palestine, and other places.

I don't know the answer to the world's political problems, but I am sure it is not for America to become the sole arbiter of world affairs. Preemptive war, in my opinion, is morally wrong regardless of who commits it — particularly when the perpetrator is the strongest nation on earth. I was as shocked by 9/11 as the next American, and felt sad for all the families touched by that tragic day's events. But even then I was convinced that the appropriate reaction for a country as powerful and as historically compassionate as ours was not to retaliate with all the force at our command but to examine ourselves and our recent history to determine why some people hated us so much that they would commit suicide in order to send us such a dramatic message.

I am not unrealistic enough to believe that expressing love and turning the other cheek would have concluded the matter. But I am idealistic enough to think that we could have found ways to spend $200 billion helping aggrieved nations and bringing the Jews and Muslims together that would have done far more to produce peace to the world than we did by mounting a war and destroying what was left of a glorious ancient civilization.

The day will come, I am confident, when the peoples of the world will find at least partial solutions to their warring madness. Globalism itself is a driving force for peace. In an era when America is China's biggest market for manufactured goods, Israel sells its flowers and produce in Japan, Germany markets its automobiles in Korea, China, and the United States, and Australia's wines, like those of France and California, are on the tables of half the world, there will be great incentives for the leaders of these nations to keep the peace in order to maintain world trade. And as the world becomes increasingly united for economic reasons, people will find more and more ways to accommodate one another's religious beliefs and practices, until one day there will be, if not a single world religion, at least a pantheon of understanding where it is possible for Christians and Buddhists, Jews and Taoists, and Hindus and Muslims to worship together.

Unfortunately I shall not live to see that day. I doubt if my children will live to see it. My grandchildren — perhaps. But meanwhile there will be great and widespread suffering, and people will continue to punish and slaughter one another in the name of justice or *jihad* because they simply do not know or understand any better way of handling their disputes.

I often think of a very obscure novel I read back in the 1970s, Thomas S. Klise's *The Last Western*. It was a big novel, but never became well known because its author was a media salesman, not a writer, and its publisher was a little-known firm called Argus Communications in Niles, Illinois. Klise was an evangelical Roman Catholic turned on to religion by Pope John XXIII and the spirit of Vatican II. Distressed by Christian history and its record of intolerance and retribution, he wrote this long story about Willie, an American Indian boy, also part Irish and part Chinese, born in the tiny town of Sandstorm, New Mexico.

ᴄ⌐ͻ

One of Willie's earliest memories was of accompanying his mother, Cool Dawn, to the little village church, where he was puzzled about the plaster figure of a man on a cross that hung above the chancel. Tugging at his mother's sleeve, he asked who the man was. She finally shushed him by saying it was "Jesus Theelord."

It worried Willie that Jesus Theelord was in bad shape — the figure was blackened by generations of candle smoke and part of the mouth had dried and fallen away. So one afternoon he sneaked into the church with a ladder and a cup of water and climbed up and poured the water into Jesus Theelord's mouth. It ran down, smearing the paint that had been applied to the wound in the statue's side, and the padre became very angry with Willie.

After an improbable career as a seminarian and then a professional baseball player, Willie became a priest and astounded everyone by becoming the first Irish-Indian-Chinese pope. He began a series of reforms in the Vatican that earned him instant and powerful enemies. At the climax of his rule he proclaimed a future "L-Day" in the world — a day of love when everyone was asked to go to anyone he or she had wronged, ask forgiveness, and make restitution. Willie himself proposed to travel to the United States and meet with a man in Illinois he had once wronged. His more sincere followers pled with him not to do it. He had many enemies, they said, who could not bear any change in their lives and would do anything to halt the progress of his papacy. But Willie traveled to Illinois in spite of their warnings.

On a winter's day, in a field covered with snow, he walked across a vast, empty space to embrace his nemesis. Shots rang out and Willie crumpled in the snow, the Christlike victim of his own dreams for peace and brotherhood.

It is an unlikely story, told first in the cadences of Richard Bach's *Jonathan Livingston Seagull* and then in the style of Kurt Vonnegut Jr. and of course with echoes of the deaths of John F. Kennedy, Robert Kennedy, and Martin Luther King Jr. But it haunts me to this day, because it is so full of my own hopes and dreams for the kingdom of God on earth, a kingdom of love and peace in a world of waste and violence.

I expect I shall go on thinking about it as long as I live.

The lack of love is so terrible. It is hard for me to imagine how anybody can live without love. I think about Judith Warner's father. Judith is a regular reviewer for the *Washington Post* "Book World." In a review of Helen Fisher's *Why We Love*, she told how her father spent years working on what he called his big *Book of Love*, intending to define love and then show people how to find it. When he died, she sorted through all his papers, hoping to find the manuscript and see if it was publishable.

All she found, she said, was a couple of old manuscripts that had been rejected by publishers back in the seventies. "And beyond that, nothing but notes — boxes and boxes and file drawers and desk drawers and closets and bookshelves and kitchen cabinets filled with notes. All expressing his passionate and prodigious hatred. Largely of me."[8]

I felt devastated for her when I read that — and for her dad, whose life must have been tragic.

Life without love is nothing — even worse than nothing. It is the same thing as life without God. John the Apostle knew what he was saying when he wrote that "God is love." They are one and the same. To discover one is to discover the other, and to miss one is to miss the other, regardless of one's protestations about either. After a long life, John must have realized it above everything he knew, that beyond all suffering, all persecution, all hardships, all misunderstanding, there is the eternal love, and that is what validates our existence. It is what, in the end, cures all our ills, mends all our quarrels, and gives us our deepest joy.

It is so sad when people can't love, when they only struggle against it instead of accepting it and wrapping themselves in it the way God intended.

I don't know what I would do if my life had been so poisoned by hate that I could not now feel an immense well of love for everything. Love is what we were made for. Not to feel it, to revel in it, and to express it is to miss the secret of everything. It is to spend life in the dark, with an unfathomable confusion rolling ceaselessly back and forth over one like the ocean in all its punishing depths. It is to die with regrets instead of happiness. It is to fail at the only thing that truly matters. It is easily the saddest thing I know.

ᴄﾉᴐ

How do I handle living in such a world?

First, by getting my own act together, and trying to live as a citizen of the kingdom in my attitude toward others. The abbot was right, in Morris West's *Clowns of God*, the only thing most of us can do, in the end, is to tend our own gardens.

Second, by praying for the world. Night and day, I beseech God to let the kingdom come, to stop the suffering of his little ones, to mend the wounds of this suffering world.

And third, by diverting myself, now that I am older, by writing and reading novels, something I rarely did before I retired.

As I said earlier, I have discovered in recent years the wonderful creations of a lot of women novelists my wife was always fond of reading, but which I, in the vanity that I had more important things to do, largely ignored. Women writers such as Barbara Delinsky, Maeve Binchy,

Rosamunde Pilcher, Anne Perry, and Elizabeth George. We both liked Patricia Cornwell for a while, until she allowed herself to be swept away into the *lingua franca* of the blasphemous younger people she was writing about, and we couldn't bear the constant atmosphere of porn and obscenity.

Anne likes for me to read to her at night, after we go to bed, and we often choose a story by Dora Saint, whose pen name is Miss Read. Saint began writing for *Punch* magazine during World War II, and went on to write dozens of novels about simple, decent folks who inhabit the little villages of the Cotswolds, that storybook area of thatched-roof houses and honey-colored stone slightly west of Oxford. One of our favorites is *The Christmas Mouse*, which we reread every December. The stories all revolve around the church, village fêtes, gossip about newcomers, and gentle romances, usually among older adults who have lost their mates. There is virtually no violence in Saint's books, and there are only occasional villains of any kind. It is a gentle, Edwardian world into which we can escape before saying our prayers and going to sleep.

Right now we are reading Elizabeth Goudge's little novel *The Middle Window*, about a girl named Judy who with her parents and fiancé in tow goes to spend the summer at an ancient house in a remote part of Scotland called Glen Suilag. There she enters into a strange relationship with the past — she thinks she has lived in the house centuries before as the mistress Judith Macdonald, and was wife to Ranald Macdonald, laird of the estate and ancestor of the present owner.

It is hardly a great novel, for Miss Goudge, who was never married, had only a romanticist's grasp of wedded life. But when she begins to describe the billowing emotions of a girl advancing into the mysteries of a life transcending her own, she is superlative. Here is a passage I marked last night, about Judy's rising and looking out the window of her big room on the morning of her birthday: "Forgetting herself in her thoughts, she leaned out of the window and greeted the day with admiring reverence. . . . Plucky little day. . . . When it had run its course one more particle of time would be bathed in light and draped in beauty; the great darkness ahead would be lessened by just so much stolen away from its horror and stored in the treasury of the past. The future, surely, was much more terrible than the past. The suffering of the past was over and done with, never to be repeated, robbed by its cessation of all its horror, existing only as the foil of joy; but the suffering of the future, that was still to be endured, a dark sea rolling on only to be conquered by the gallant little days that met and accepted it, endured it, and left it behind them robbed of its sting."[9]

This clear and simple paragraph might well be an epigraph for this book, *Winter Soulstice*. Goudge obviously loved memories, and regarded the past as something wonderfully controllable in comparison with the uncertainties of a tumultuous present and the threatening future.

Mentioning *Winter Soulstice* reminds me once again of Rosamunde Pilcher's *Winter Solstice*, one of our night reads a couple of years ago. Pilcher's books are almost invariably set in one of two locations, the far southwest of England or the rural and village areas of Scotland. The books are filled with the simple, largely uncomplicated lives of very ordinary people, into whose emotions Pilcher taps with the skill of a neurosurgeon. They are very *civilized* books. People think and act within a framework of thoughtfulness, restraint, and compassion, so that Pilcher's writings are a wonderful antidote to the normal madness of our lives in modern America. Her characters inhabit a setting where things are reasonably adjustable and people can change their circumstances to improve their chances of happiness, the way the heroine of *The Shell Seekers* does after her husband dies and her children are always on at her about selling his paintings and making their existence more comfortable.

Of course there is an element of escape in our reading such books. Aren't most works of fiction written as vehicles of escape? Perhaps some aren't — James Joyce's *Finnegans Wake* and Samuel Beckett's *Murphy* and *Malloy* novels come to mind — but most undoubtedly are. Even Saul Bellow's and Thomas Pynchon's and Joyce Carol Oates's stories, which have a hard, exploratory side to them as well.

And I realize there is also an aspect of escape in my turning now to the writing of fiction, something I rarely indulged myself in past years (the Jessie novels were an exception). Jonathan Edwards, the great eighteenth-century New England divine who is still considered America's most important theologian, would not permit himself to read novels, even though he wanted to read those of Joseph Fielding in order to improve his own style of writing. For years, I thought of Edwards and agreed with his self-imposed restriction lest I fritter away valuable time on non-serious writing. I was also mindful of Graham Greene's distinction between his great novels, such as *The Power and the Glory* and *The Heart of the Matter*, and the stories he called "entertainments," such as *The Third Man* and *Our Man in Havana*. But I was too busy even to permit myself the writing of more entertaining books. Now, I confess, I relish the time I spend creating the works of fiction that seem to flood my mind — and wonder if they won't in the end be more important than my other writings.

I have already alluded to the one serious book I would still like to write — the one called *God by Any Other Name: The Deity of the Coming Global Religion*. But when that is accomplished, I think I shall feel discharged of all responsibilities and free to enjoy myself in any fictional pieces I can manage. Heaven only knows what those are likely to be, although there are two series of works I can envision, one involving additions to the Jessie novels I have already written — I have long thought I would write one about Jessie in Hollywood — and the other consisting of sequels to *Maggie Bowles: The Mystery of the Marigold Turtle*. Maggie's story is about the experiences of a woman minister in a resort setting inspired by Mackinac Island, Michigan, where Anne and I spent so many summers at the Little Stone Church. I wrote it originally as a quiet, simple narrative called *A Summer on Marigold Island*. But now I am turning it into a mystery story because it is so difficult today to find publishers for books without more aggressive plots.

Still, I am feeling delightfully "undriven" since I retired, and at liberty to do just about anything I feel like doing. (A friend sent me an e-mail about "the undriven life," as opposed to the kind of existence advocated by Rick Warren's extraordinarily popular *The Purpose Driven Life*.) It was a rare-enough occasion, when I was at the prime of my working career, to get caught up on things and feel that I had an evening or a weekend in which I might simply enjoy myself. Now this appears to be a more or less permanent condition. Yet I am rarely at loose ends. There are always projects suggesting — even urging — themselves on me. It is a good feeling, perhaps not unlike that of a movie star who has turned in a good performance or two and can relax, glance over all the scripts that pour in, and select one merely for the fun of it, not because it is necessary to her career.

⌒ↄ

One thing I do notice in these latter years is how long my prayer list has become. C. S. Lewis once said that that is the wretched thing about prayer lists: the older one gets and the more people one knows, the longer the list becomes. That is certainly true in my case.

Right now I am remembering each day a friend in Texas who has had serious hand surgery, the father of a friend in Alabama who was taken to hospital with a heart problem, a friend's three-year-old nephew in Arkansas who has been diagnosed with inoperable cancer of the brain stem, a friend whose long-term bout with diabetes has now made her blind, another friend whose husband has recently died, a brother-in-law who broke his hip, his wife who is working beyond her sell-by date because she can't afford to buy her own health insurance, a woman I met at a local hospital who was just going on chemotherapy for cancer and is especially worried because her father and sister both died of cancer during the last two years, a neighbor who has had a foot operation, an old friend who has just had a prostatectomy, a minister friend who is feeling depressed about the churches he has been assigned to serve, another minister friend, still relatively young, whose Parkinson's disease is threatening his career, a doctor friend who has cancer, a minister friend who is undergoing stem-cell replacement for multiple myeloma, a singer friend who has a growth on his vocal cords that the doctors can't diagnose, a friend who needs heart surgery but whose esophagus has been rejecting the camera they have tried to feed down into his chest, an editor friend whose husband is older and has chronic health problems, a friend who was in a car crash, has lost one eye, and is in danger of losing another, a sister-in-law who has been having a series of TIAs and isn't allowed to blow her nose because of a hematoma on the brain, the husband of a woman I met in Wal-Mart who said he has been in and out of the hospital for a year and a half with an ailment of the pancreas and liver that the doctors haven't been able to diagnose, a minister who has UIP, usual interstitial pneumonia, an untreatable lung infection that the doctors think will be fatal within a few months, and, of course, my wife and our sons and their wives, and now, without fail, our little granddaughters, Ellie and Chloe, who are both under two years of age.

The case of the minister with a lung infection is interesting. I met him on Mackinac Island over a year ago, and when I retired from being the minister there he was invited to conduct services and perform the weddings for three weeks. I heard from friends on the island that he was having a very difficult time breathing, and had to pause to rest even when walking a short distance to the church. About to enter the hospital myself for lung surgery, I telephoned and talked with him about his problem. At that point, it had not been fully diagnosed. All he knew was that he had a serious infection that was impairing his breathing.

Remembering a friend in Princeton, New Jersey, who had what sounded like a similar problem after handling pressure-treated wood, I asked Bob (I must give him at least part of his name) if he was a woodworker. Yes, he said, he had recently completed a big jungle gym for his grandchildren that was made of treated wood. I put him in touch with my friend in New Jersey, and for a while it sounded as if the woodworking might be his problem.

Then he went to the clinic at the University of Michigan, where the doctors biopsied his lungs and announced that he had UIP.

A day or two before I had heard about their decision, my agent-friend Kathleen Niendorff in Austin, Texas, told me about a miraculous thing that happened at a conference where one of her clients was speaking. He had been diagnosed with advanced cancer and given a short time to live. Yet he was determined to fulfill his speaking obligation. At the conference, a small woman named Sandy came up to him and said he looked as if he didn't feel well. He told her that he didn't have long to live.

"May I pray for you?" she asked, and reached up — he was tall and she was not — to place her hand on his forehead.

As she stood there praying for him, he felt a strange electric current pass through his body, and immediately began to feel better. When he went to the doctor a few days later, there was no sign of his cancer. It had completely vanished.

I asked Bob if it was all right for me to get in touch with Sandy in his behalf. He had no objection. So I telephoned Kathleen and asked for Sandy's phone number. I called and left a message, and Sandy returned it. I told her about Bob and said that she appeared to be a special conduit of grace and I would like to put the two of them in touch. If she decided that she needed to see Bob in person, I said, I would gladly pay for her plane ticket to Michigan.

Sandy told me that she had a little group of friends who met for inter-cessory prayer every Saturday morning and they would begin by praying for Bob in the group. When she notified Bob of their intention, he and his wife, Margie, called their minister and his wife to join them for prayer at the time on Saturday morning when the group was praying. That has been going on now for about three months. Bob has not thrown off the infection, but he is getting better. His breathing measurements have improved, and he feels much better than he did before. The doctors are baffled. People with UIP are not supposed to get better at all but normally suffer a steady decline.

Two days ago, I had a letter from Margie enclosing a magazine article about a woman with big-time back problems who had multiple operations and was still suffering so badly that her life was completely disrupted. She had been to doctor after doctor, and had even attended a pain clinic in New York, but nobody seemed to be able to alleviate her awful suffering. Then a friend persuaded her to go to a healing conference with Francis McNutt, the Roman Catholic priest who has written several books on faith healing.

Francis, whom I met years ago when I was a professor at Vanderbilt, asked two women to pray with her. They were joined by a third woman the others didn't know. This woman knelt and placed her hand on the woman's back where the pain was most intense. Suddenly an electric current passed through her body and the pain began to subside. The woman asked her to stand. As she pressed on her body and was told where the pain was now, she held the place again, and once more the current rippled through her body like little shock waves.

Joyfully the woman announced that her pain was gone. She hugged the two women who had first come to pray with her. Then she turned to hug the third woman. But the third woman was gone. She had left without even telling them her name. Now without pain for more than two years, the woman made an all-out effort to find the third person, the one whose touch had brought healing. But no one at Francis McNutt's organization had ever heard of her. The woman is convinced that she was an angel.

As I read this account in Margie's letter, I remembered our friend Wilma Ringstrom, who for many years was president of an organization called Religion in Drama and the Other Arts. I spoke for the organization several times. Wilma's husband was a vice president of the A&P Company and they lived in St. Louis. When he was fired in a company reorganization, we lived through the news with Wilma, and kept them both in our prayers for months.

The last time I saw Wilma, at a meeting in Nashville, she told an incredible story about having inoperable stomach cancer. She had gone to the hospital for surgery, but the doctors had taken one look at her stomach and closed her back up, saying there was no point in operating. She was in enormous pain. Even heavy doses of morphine didn't quell the suffering. During that horrible night in the hospital, a strangely attired woman entered Wilma's room and asked in a very soothing voice how she was doing. Wilma said she felt awful. The woman was a large African American, perhaps from the Caribbean, and wore a colorful turban. She asked Wilma's permission to give her a massage, saying that it would help her to sleep. Wilma gave her consent and the woman began kneading her body. As she kneaded, the pain began to subside, and eventually Wilma, who was exhausted, fell into a deep sleep.

The next morning, she felt great. There was no sign of the pain. "I'm going home," she announced. The doctors and nurses advised against it, but Wilma was determined, so she dressed and left the hospital.

When Wilma was x-rayed a few days later, there were no signs of the cancer. Her doctor couldn't believe it. But Wilma stood before him happy and pain free.

Like the woman who tried to find the person who touched her at Francis McNutt's meeting, Wilma searched for the strange woman who had come into her hospital room and given her a massage. She asked the nurses at the hospital, but none of them knew of such a woman and said she certainly wasn't a member of their staff.

A few weeks later, Wilma was speaking at a meeting in St. Louis when she saw the woman with the turban enter the back of the hall. The woman smiled radiantly at her, and Wilma could hardly wait to finish her talk and find the woman to thank her. But again the woman disappeared, and Wilma never saw her again.

She too believed she had been healed by an angel.

Here too the coalescence is occurring — memories, body, friends and associates, spiritual life in general. Prayer and healing have more weight for me than they ever had before. Some days I think I exist now merely to pray for others, the way our friend Sister Anastasia did at the Benedictine convent in Nashville. Sister spent most of her life teaching music in the convent school. But when she got too old to teach, she was retired to praying and spent her days and evenings at the altar in the chapel of the motherhouse. I suspect sometimes that I too am retired to praying. My whole being is concentrated in my concern for others. It seems to be a fitting end — and a welcome unification — to a long and varied career.

ↄ

Which brings me back to a recurring theme of my life — the appearance of Gabriel and what my wife and son saw that night in the hospital chapel in Detroit. There are things going on in this world that are beyond our knowing or understanding. I have always believed that there is a transcendental dimension at work in our lives, even when we aren't aware of it. And the most important thing we can do for ourselves is to practice being aware, to become more and more sensitive to messengers of God coming and going right under our noses.

For example, I just had an e-mail from Margie, the wife of Bob, the minister with UIP, saying that he continues to improve and can now spend most of the day without supplemental oxygen. Then she mentioned something else. Last Saturday morning, when the prayer group in Austin was praying for Bob, and he and Margie and two friends were praying at their home in Michigan, she and Bob looked out and saw a dozen bluebirds flying around their window.

"We don't have bluebirds in Michigan in the winter," said Margie, "and certainly not a dozen of them at one time."

They were convinced that the birds, which continued to fly around their backyard for several minutes, were a sign of special grace.

I think so too.

I am not a religious fanatic. In fact, the older I get, the more suspicious I am of most religion as something humanly concocted, not divinely revealed. Maybe there was a divine seed in it back at the time of its origin — some sense of the numinous that then got translated into human form.

But afterward, like everything else, it became polluted by earthly ideas and finite understandings until it was nothing like the image or event that produced it.

Yet I am totally convinced of the ultimate spirituality of life itself — that we live and move and have our being in God, even when we are unaware that we're doing it. And part of the spirituality of our elder years has to do with an increasing recognition of this. I am sure this is why I am so happy to be in the latter period of my life, when I can see everything coming together so beautifully.

I love what the chaos theorists are doing with computer projections. They can relate the most apparently disparate facts by extrapolating from them to the future and showing how they are all interrelated in beautiful patterns, regardless of how they appear to us. For example, take such distant and — we think — unrelated occurrences as a bird's singing outside your window, a wave washing ashore on Martha's Vineyard, and a woman's beating her wash on the rocks in a remote province of China. When these are fed into supercomputers as digitalized information, the computers produce a series of graceful-looking graphs. The lines link the occurrences with countless others, as though they were all being observed from millions of miles in space, where the relationships would doubtless appear more obvious. We are simply too close to everything to understand this except by faith.

Now everything appears to be grandly merging for me — memories, work, play, body, the books I read, numinous experiences, all of it. I can no longer feel or make hard-and-fast distinctions between waking and dreams, friends and enemies, body and soul. The old categories have all started collapsing into one another, and life is becoming increasingly unified. Everything coalesces like an organism repairing itself by filling in the blank spaces until it is totally whole, yet related to every other whole in the universe.

It is uncanny. I feel as if I am somehow melding with God and becoming an indistinguishable part of the totality of all that is. It is happening more and more every day, and my heart is filled with an indescribable joy.

I marvel at the sense of acceptance I discern in my own being. I have a profound trust that this amazing process is good, and that it has to do with God. I know that when it is complete, my happiness will not recognize any boundaries. It is as if I am daily breaking loose from my chrysalis — I can almost hear it groaning and cracking all around me — and am about to fly away with the incredible lightness of a butterfly, and be caught in the wonderful updrafts and downdrafts of eternity. I experience what the French psychoanalyst Jacques Lacan has called *jouissance* — "extravagant, unreasonable joy."

I don't feel it all the time. I admit that there are days when my soul is heavy and sullen, especially when I contemplate the suffering and adversities of people around the globe and then become upset with world leaders and authorities who have the most power to alleviate these, yet make no effort to do so. But I'm feeling it more and more, and the sense of it is always there, just inches away, so that I can slip into it almost at will.

It is a gift. I recognize that. I didn't make it happen. It isn't the result of any wisdom I possess or any process I control. On the contrary, it is merely something that has happened to me, for which I can take absolutely no credit. So I bow my head and thank God for it. And I pray that others may feel it too — that I am not the only one — and that this book may help some readers to recognize a similar process occurring in their own lives.

∽

There is a little story that sums up everything. It appeared years ago in *Reader's Digest* — one of those "Life in the United States" stories, I think. I have told it so often that I cannot any longer be sure that the wording is correct. But I remember the gist perfectly.

One day an old man in Florida took his little grandson fishing off a dock. All day, the little boy questioned his grandpa about things — why it rains, where birds go when they die, whether fish feel the hooks that impale them, why the leaves change colors in the fall — and the grandfather tried patiently and lovingly to answer every query.

At twilight, the grandfather said it was time to go home. So they removed the bait from their hooks and were preparing their tackle to leave, when the little boy looked up at his grandfather and asked one more question.

"Grandpa," he said, "does anybody ever see God?"

The old man looked out at the deepening hues of the setting sun. Then he looked in the face of the little boy, whom he loved beyond everything else in the world. He thought of the wonderful day they had just spent together. His eyes filled with tears.

"Son," he said, "it's getting so I hardly see anything else."

That's the way it is for me. I suspect it's that way for everybody when we grow older and become more sensitive to everything around us. It is the gift that comes with age. And when it comes, we find that it's what we've been waiting for all our lives.

What did Jesus say to the thief on the cross? "Today you shall be with me in paradise."

Now there's a tear in my eye, because I realize that I'm already in paradise!

Notes

1. Frederick Buechner, *The Alphabet of Grace* (New York: Seabury Press, 1970), 3–4.

2. D. H. Lawrence, *The Rainbow* (New York: Viking, 1961), 1–2.

3. Henry Miller, *The Wisdom of the Heart* (New York: New Directions, 1960), 22.

4. Samuel Beckett, *Krapp's Last Tape and Other Pieces* (New York: Grove Press, n.d.), 21.

5. Madeleine L'Engle, *Two-Part Invention* (New York: Harper & Row, 1989), 184.

6. Browning Ware, *Diary of a Modern Pilgrim* (Austin, Tex.: Imago Dei Publications, 2003), 219.

7. Ibid., 214.

8. Judith Warner, review of *Why We Love* by Helen Fisher, *Washington Post Book World*, February 8, 2004, 3.

9. Elizabeth Goudge, *The Middle Window* (New York: Pyramid Books, 1973), 120.

Acknowledgments

Our lives are so totally interfused with those of others that it is impossible to think of anything we do as solely ours. Certainly that is the case with this book, which is as much the product of other persons and their effect on me as it is of anything I might have brought to it on my own. Many of those persons are obvious — parents, teachers, students, spouse, children, heroes, favorite authors, colleagues, parishioners, friends, even enemies (who are only friends that haven't been converted). I have alluded to some of them, but for every one I have mentioned there are at least ten, a dozen, or a hundred more who regretfully could not be included because of lack of space. I hope they know who they are, and that I have not failed, across the years, to signal to them in significant and memorable ways how much they have meant to me. Even though their names may be omitted here, I would not, apart from them, begin to be who I am or to think and behave as I do.

Also, every book, in its ultimate birthing, requires numerous midwives — readers who decide on its merits, editors whose work is almost always best when least apparent, computerists and printers and binders who convert the dream into hard reality, advertising and marketing people who blow their figurative trumpets before the nearly finished product, sales representatives who commend it in various venues, clerks and other personnel in those venues who actually handle individual copies of the book, and finally, of course, the readers themselves, without whom there would be no point in writing. Each of these is immeasurably important, and no book could ever exist without them.

I am particularly grateful, in this instance, to Jean Blomquist, my efficient and sometimes necessarily ruthless copyeditor, and Roy M. Carlisle, senior editor of the Crossroad Publishing Company, who went far beyond the usual call of duty to cajole and prod me toward the producing of a book that, in the end, represented his vision as well as mine of what *Winter Soulstice* should become. Thanks, dear and patient friends, for helping me to express what I really couldn't have expressed half so well without you!

About the Author

John Killinger has had a distinguished career as a churchman, professor, and author. Holder of a Ph.D. in theology from Princeton University and another Ph.D. in literature from the University of Kentucky, he taught preaching, worship, and literature at Vanderbilt Divinity School from 1965 to 1980. He has also taught as a visiting professor at the University of Chicago, City College of New York, Princeton Seminary, and Claremont School of Theology, and was Distinguished Professor of Religion and Culture at Samford University in Birmingham, Alabama.

Ordained as a Baptist minister at the age of eighteen, he left teaching for a decade in the 1980s to be senior minister of the First Presbyterian Church in Lynchburg, Virginia. He then became senior minister of the First Congregational Church of Los Angeles, the oldest English-speaking congregation in that city. Since leaving Samford University in 1996 he has also served as minister of the Little Stone Church on Mackinac Island, Michigan.

Dr. Killinger has written more than fifty books, on subjects ranging from Hemingway and the Theater of the Absurd to prayers, preaching, and biblical commentary as well as fiction. He has also served on the editorial boards of *Christian Ministry*, *Pulpit Digest*, and the Library of Distinctive Sermons.

John and his wife, Anne (also an author), love reading, writing, travel, theater, and hiking. Their rambling home is on the outskirts of Warrenton, Virginia, halfway between the nation's capital and the Blue Ridge Mountains.

A Word from the Editor

Ageing is a complicated, challenging, and even frustrating reality for many of us. We want to do it well, but we live in a culture where it is definitely more acceptable — if not required — to "stay" young than it is to age gracefully. It seems that nothing worth having, if you listen to any media, is obtainable unless we are young, or at least look young, and beautiful. How can any of us stay young? What is this preoccupation about anyway? It makes no sense and it is impossible, and yet enormous amounts of energy and money are expended in pursuing an unreachable goal of at least looking young even if we can't slow down the passing of the years. I know this struggle intimately, as a white male in his fifties who has a chronic disease (Type II diabetes) but who wants to stay healthy, fit, and young at heart. But John Killinger, and his lovely wife, Anne, seem to have leapt over my banal struggles to stay "young" and healthy, some of which have been embarrassingly well documented in my periodic running reflections for many to see.

I remember a time when I was traveling to the area where the Killingers lived and they opened up one of their lovely guest rooms to me in their spacious home in Virginia. One morning I had gone out for a run. It was a cool September day, and autumn had come to the East Coast with a drop in temperature and a bit of rain. As I was jogging along a country road (with furious clanging by large machines in a housing development in the midst of the verdant landscape) I thought about how generously and easily they both lived in the world and in their selves. There was a certain seamlessness in how they wore faith, joy, and individuality during these golden years. It reminded me of the *Chronicles of Narnia* and *The Great Divorce* by C. S. Lewis, both fictional narratives wherein we eventually meet characters who glow from within and who seem to be ageless. John and Anne are like that. Certainly they are both authentically themselves and at the same time they are very much at peace with themselves and the temporal world in which all of us live. I am not like that; I am still clanging along — like those large machines in the housing development across the road — trying to make everything fit and trying too hard to juggle too many demands and desires. It wasn't exactly an epiphany but it was an impression that sank into my soul.

I must admit, though, that this book was another lesson in how an editor's vision is sometimes at slight variance with an author's vision. John is more content to tell the story and let the readers find their own meaning. I wanted more philosophy and reflection, clearly because I wanted John to provide pastoral care in this book as he does in person. We finally began to strike a balance between the two visions. But I think you will find that John (and Anne's) story has a way of "working" on you. It begins to reveal itself in the way that John and Anne have lived their lives, made the decisions they have made, and supremely in how they have "enjoyed" their journey. This does not mean, of course, that John has not run up against brick walls, bounced off obstacles in the path, or disagreed quite intensely with those who have deigned to thwart him in his ministry. In spite of all of that, he and Anne do indeed enjoy themselves and enjoy their family, their work, their travels. It is this capacity for enjoyment that keeps haunting me. And it haunts this book. It haunts me because I don't do "enjoyment" very well. Again C. S. Lewis comes to mind because in a hundred different ways and in a dozen different books he gives us a glimpse of how true enjoyment of life and of simple life tasks can be deeply spiritual. That was a new thought to me when I first encountered it in Lewis's writings during my college years, and it surprised me. My adopted form of conservative Christian practice and belief definitely did not promote enjoyment in life or of life.

And it haunts this book because the sad truth is that the relationship between enjoyment and spirituality that is very evident in this story still surprises me. But I am hoping that you have learned about this dimension of spirituality much sooner than I, and thus you will have recognized how valuable a memoir of this type really is. John's actual description of the lives lived and his poetic language work hand in glove to make this an "enjoyable" read. In that experience of enjoyment you will have come a few steps closer to maintaining the balance of a life lived with the full knowledge that God is active in human affairs (whether you believe it or not) and that God's presence can be the "fullness of joy" that most of us miss. In the many versions of the Baltimore Catechism (the first was published in 1891) the references to "happiness" with God as our purpose in life and in the life beyond are many and varied and that theme continues throughout all of the revisions and expansions of the Catechism. And there is the famous line in the Westminster Shorter Catechism by Matthew Henry about the chief end of Man which is "to Glorify God, and to Enjoy Him forever." (Excuse the sexist language, but this was written in 1648). I don't ever remember hearing the words "God," "happiness," and "enjoyment" in the same sentence in my early years as a Christian. I am not saying that it wasn't uttered, but I am saying that I didn't *hear* it. So I want you to read this remarkable memoir and see (and hear) that joy and wisdom join hands in the Christian life. I want this book to help you understand that you really can enjoy the second half of life; in fact you are encouraged to enjoy the second half of life. The Killingers certainly have, and so can we. And in that enjoyment we can find our own unique form of peace and spirituality.

Roy M. Carlisle
Senior Editor

Of Related Interest

John Killinger
TEN THINGS I LEARNED WRONG
FROM A CONSERVATIVE CHURCH

John Killinger warmly relates the story of his salvation from an abusive father by the kindly people of his local Baptist church in rural Kentucky. Part memoir, part theological reflection, this story will be of help to many who wish to remain faithful to the Lord, but struggle with the strict tenets of biblical fundamentalism.

0-8245-2011-4, $21.95 hardcover

Paula D'Arcy
SACRED THRESHOLD
Crossing the Inner Barrier to a Deeper Love

Includes the author's own story of her relationship with Morrie Schwartz of *Tuesdays with Morrie* and other stories of healing and love.

Something new and unanticipated happened when I read Paula's *Sacred Threshold*. She not only brought me to the threshold with which I separate myself from God; she opened me up to the startling discovery of who I am. This book is a must-read for all who want to know the Genuine.

–Rev. John Blackwell, Ph.D., author of *Noonday Demon*

0-8245-2278-8, $17.95 hardcover

crossroad

Of Related Interest

Jean Colgan Gould
FORTY YEARS SINCE MY LAST CONFESSION
A Memoir

The newest in the Crossroad series of Catholic memoirs is a richly poetic, intuitive story of how one woman, a bright and headstrong seeker of spiritual truth, finds her way back to the Catholic faith of her childhood. Against the backdrop of stormy political church battles over issues such as feminism and social ethics, her story is about the interior process all of us experience when we find ourselves outsiders and strangers trying to build a home and a community.

"This is a wonderfully evocative, beautifully written book, and a great read." — William A. Barry, S.J., author of *Letting God Come Close*

0-8245-2144-7, $18.95 paperback

C. McNair Wilson
RAISED IN CAPTIVITY
How to Survive (and Thrive in) a Religiously Addicted Family

Actor and humorist McNair Wilson is back with his first new book in over two decades. In this hilarious memoir, he pokes fun at everything from Sunday School to strict sexual mores.

Wilson is a former Disney Imagineer who's currently on the road forty weeks a year giving motivational speeches on "Imaginuity," his self-titled creative brainstorming process. Patricia Fripp, past president of the National Speakers Association, has said this of his seminars: "McNair Wilson's talk on Creativity is one of the most dynamic, profound, and enjoyable talks I have ever heard."

0-8245-2118-8, $16.95 paperback

crossroad

Of Related Interest

Mani L. Bhaumik
CODE NAME GOD
The Spiritual Odyssey of a Man of Science

Born and raised in an impoverished area of India, Dr. Bhaumik went
on to become a physicist famous as the co-inventor of excimer laser
technology, the miracle behind LASIK eye surgery that has improved
the lives of thousands of people. But fame and success weren't enough.

"One day, I was sipping a glass of Château Lafit Rothschild wine with
Hollywood celebrities and enjoying the life of a self-made scientific
entrepreneur with a stint on *Lifestyles of the Rich and Famous*. The
next, I was on my knees before the enormous emptiness of that existence and searching for answers to questions I hadn't asked for a long
time. However many (or few) houses I was destined to own in the
future, I did not want to feel again so completely alone in them. However many lovely islands I might be privileged to gaze at, I wanted to
know that their reality owed its existence to the same force that had
shaped my own being."

In *Code Name God*, Bhaumik offers us his remarkable rags-to-riches
story, his understanding of the true nature of science, and his vision
of spirituality as that which gives meaning to our lives.

0-8245-2281-8, $17.95 hardcover

Please support your local bookstore,
or call 1-800-707-0670 for Customer Service.

For a free catalog, write us at

THE CROSSROAD PUBLISHING COMPANY
16 Penn Plaza – 481 Eighth Avenue, Suite 1550
New York, NY 10001

Visit our website at
www.crossroadpublishing.com
All prices subject to change.

crossroad